T0259356

Cerebrovascular Diseases: Controversies and Challenges

Editor

WILLIAM J. POWERS

NEUROLOGIC CLINICS

www.neurologic.theclinics.com

Consulting Editor
RANDOLPH W. EVANS

May 2015 • Volume 33 • Number 2

ELSEVIER

1600 John F. Kennedy Boulevard • Suite 1800 • Philadelphia, Pennsylvania, 19103-2899

http://www.theclinics.com

NEUROLOGIC CLINICS Volume 33, Number 2
May 2015 ISSN 0733-8619, ISBN-13: 978-0-323-37611-2

Editor: Joanne Husovski
Developmental editor: Donald Mumford

© **2015 Elsevier Inc. All rights reserved.**

This periodical and the individual contributions contained in it are protected under copyright by Elsevier, and the following terms and conditions apply to their use:

Photocopying
Single photocopies of single articles may be made for personal use as allowed by national copyright laws. Permission of the Publisher and payment of a fee is required for all other photocopying, including multiple or systematic copying, copying for advertising or promotional purposes, resale, and all forms of document delivery. Special rates are available for educational institutions that wish to make photocopies for non-profit educational classroom use. For information on how to seek permission visit www.elsevier.com/permissions or call: (+44) 1865 843830 (UK)/(+1) 215 239 3804 (USA).

Derivative Works
Subscribers may reproduce tables of contents or prepare lists of articles including abstracts for internal circulation within their institutions. Permission of the Publisher is required for resale or distribution outside the institution. Permission of the Publisher is required for all other derivative works, including compilations and translations (please consult www.elsevier.com/permissions).

Electronic Storage or Usage
Permission of the Publisher is required to store or use electronically any material contained in this periodical, including any article or part of an article (please consult www.elsevier.com/permissions). Except as outlined above, no part of this publication may be reproduced, stored in a retrieval system or transmitted in any form or by any means, electronic, mechanical, photocopying, recording or otherwise, without prior written permission of the Publisher.

Notice
No responsibility is assumed by the Publisher for any injury and/or damage to persons or property as a matter of products liability, negligence or otherwise, or from any use or operation of any methods, products, instructions or ideas contained in the material herein. Because of rapid advances in the medical sciences, in particular, independent verification of diagnoses and drug dosages should be made.

Although all advertising material is expected to conform to ethical (medical) standards, inclusion in this publication does not constitute a guarantee or endorsement of the quality or value of such product or of the claims made of it by its manufacturer.

Neurologic Clinics (ISSN 0733-8619) is published quarterly by Elsevier Inc., 360 Park Avenue South, New York, NY 10010–1710. Months of issue are February, May, August, and November. Periodicals postage paid at New York, NY, and additional mailing offices. Subscription prices are $300.00 per year for US individuals, $517.00 per year for US institutions, $145.00 per year for US students, $375.00 per year for Canadian individuals, $627.00 per year for Canadian institutions, $415.00 per year for international individuals, $627.00 per year for international institutions, and $210.00 for Canadian and foreign students/residents. To receive student/resident rate, orders must be accompanied by name of affiliated institution, date of term, and the *signature* of program/residency coordinator on institution letterhead. Orders will be billed at individual rate until proof of status is received. Foreign air speed delivery is included in all *Clinics* subscription prices. All prices are subject to change without notice. **POSTMASTER:** Send address changes to *Neurologic Clinics*, Elsevier Health Sciences Division, Subscription Customer Service, 3251 Riverport Lane, Maryland Heights, MO 63043. **Customer Service: Telephone: 1-800-654-2452 (U.S. and Canada); 314-447-8871 (outside U.S. and Canada). Fax: 314-447-8029. E-mail: journalscustomerservice-usa@elsevier.com (for print support); journalsonlinesupport-usa@elsevier.com (for online support).**

Reprints. For copies of 100 or more of articles in this publication, please contact the Commercial Reprints Department, Elsevier Inc., 360 Park Avenue South, New York, New York, 10010-1710; Tel.: +1-212-633-3874; Fax: +1-212-633-3820, and E-mail: reprints@elsevier.com.

Neurologic Clinics is also published in Spanish by Nueva Editorial Interamericana S.A., Mexico City, Mexico.

Neurologic Clinics is covered in *Current Contents/Clinical Medicine, MEDLINE/PubMed (Index Medicus), EMBASE/Excerpta Medica, and PsycINFO, and ISI/BIOMED.*

Contributors

CONSULTING EDITOR

RANDOLPH W. EVANS, MD
Clinical Professor of Neurology, Baylor College of Medicine, Houston, Texas

EDITOR

WILLIAM J. POWERS, MD
H. Houston Merritt Distinguished Professor and Chair, Department of Neurology, University of North Carolina School of Medicine, Chapel Hill, North Carolina

AUTHORS

CLOTILDE BALUCANI, MD, PhD
Research Assistant Professor, State University of New York Downstate Medical Center and Stroke Center, Brooklyn, New York

LEO BONATI, MD
Head, Acute Stroke Unit, Department of Neurology, Stroke Center, University Hospital Basel, Basel, Switzerland

CHARLOTTE CORDONNIER, MD, PhD
Department of Neurology, University of Lille, UDSL, CHU Lille, Lille, France

RENAN DOMINGUES, MD
Department of Neurology, University of Lille, UDSL, CHU Lille, Lille, France; CAPES Foundation, Ministry of Education, Brasilia-DF, Brazil

STEFAN T. ENGELTER, MD
Department of Neurology and Stroke Center, University Hospital Basel; Neurorehabilitation Unit, Felix Platter Hospital, University Center for Medicine of Aging and Rehabilitation, Basel, Switzerland

REZA JAHAN, MD
Professor, Division of Interventional Neuroradiology, Department of Radiology, David Geffen School of Medicine at University of California Los Angeles, Los Angeles, California

SEBY JOHN, MD
Vascular Neurology Fellow, Cerebrovascular Center, Cleveland Clinic, Cleveland, Ohio

J. DEDRICK JORDAN, MD, PhD
Departments of Neurology and Neurosurgery, University of North Carolina at Chapel Hill School of Medicine, Chapel Hill, North Carolina

CHANDNI KALARIA, MD
Department of Neurology, University of Maryland School of Medicine, Baltimore, Maryland

IRENE KATZAN, MD
Director, Neurological Institute Center for Outcomes Research and Evaluation, Cleveland Clinic, Cleveland, Ohio

DAVID M. KENT, MD, MS
Professor of Medicine, Predictive Analytics and Comparative Effectiveness Center, Institute for Clinical Research and Health Policy Studies, Tufts Medical Center, Tufts University School of Medicine, Boston, Massachusetts

CHELSEA S. KIDWELL, MD
Professor of Neurology and Medical Imaging; Vice Chair of Research, Department of Neurology, University of Arizona, Tucson, Arizona

STEVEN KITTNER, MD, MPH
Professor, Department of Neurology, University of Maryland School of Medicine; Department of Neurology, Baltimore Veterans Administration Medical Center, Baltimore, Maryland

STEVEN R. LEVINE, MD, FAHA, FAAN, FANA
Professor of Neurology and Emergency Medicine, State University of New York Downstate Medical Center and Stroke Center, The Kings County Hospital Center, Brooklyn, New York

PHILIPPE A. LYRER, MD
Department of Neurology and Stroke Center, University Hospital Basel, Basel, Switzerland

ADRIAN MARCHIDANN, MD
Assistant Professor of Neurology, State University of New York Downstate Medical Center and Stroke Center, The Kings County Hospital Center, Brooklyn, New York

J.P. MOHR, MD, MS
Daniel Sciarra Professor of Neurology, Department of Neurology, Doris and Stanley Tananbaum Stroke Center, Neurological Institute, Columbia University Medical Center, New York, New York

KATHRYN A. MORBITZER, PharmD
Division of Practice Advancement and Clinical Education, University of North Carolina Eshelman School of Pharmacy, University of North Carolina at Chapel Hill, Chapel Hill, North Carolina

WILLIAM J. POWERS, MD
H. Houston Merritt Distinguished Professor and Chair, Department of Neurology, University of North Carolina School of Medicine, Chapel Hill, North Carolina

DENISE H. RHONEY, PharmD, FCCP, FCCM, FNCS
Division of Practice Advancement and Clinical Education, University of North Carolina Eshelman School of Pharmacy, University of North Carolina at Chapel Hill, Chapel Hill, North Carolina

COSTANZA ROSSI, MD, PhD
Department of Neurology, University of Lille, UDSL, CHU Lille, Lille, France

J. DAVID SPENCE, MD, FRCPC, FAHA
Director, Stroke Prevention and Atherosclerosis Research Centre, Robarts Research Institute; Professor of Neurology and Clinical Pharmacology, Western University, London, Ontario, Canada

CHRISTOPHER TRAENKA, MD
Department of Neurology and Stroke Center, University Hospital Basel, Basel, Switzerland

ALEXANDER VON HESSLING, MD
Department of Radiology, Neuroradiology and Stroke Center, University Hospital Basel, Basel, Switzerland

BENJAMIN S. WESSLER, MD
Cardiology Fellow, Predictive Analytics and Comparative Effectiveness Center, Institute for Clinical Research and Health Policy Studies, Tufts Medical Center, Tufts University School of Medicine; Division of Cardiology, Tufts Medical Center, Boston, Massachusetts

SHADI YAGHI, MD
Vascular Neurology Fellow, Department of Neurology, Doris and Stanley Tananbaum Stroke Center, Neurological Institute, Columbia University Medical Center, New York, New York

ALLYSON ZAZULIA, MD
Associate Professor of Neurology and Radiology; Associate Dean for Continuing Medical Education, Washington University School of Medicine, St Louis, Missouri

Contents

thrombolysis in patients with CAD-related stroke. Because intravenous-thrombolyzed CAD patients might not recover as well as other stroke patients, acute endovascular treatment is an alternative. Regarding the choice of antithrombotic agents, this article discusses the findings of 4 meta-analyses across observational data, the current status of 3 randomized controlled trials, and arguments and counterarguments favoring anticoagulants over antiplatelets. Furthermore, the role of stenting and surgery is addressed.

With modern intensive medical therapy, the risk of ipsilateral stroke in patients with asymptomatic carotid stenosis (ACS) is below the risk of either carotid stenting or endarterectomy. Routine intervention for ACS is therefore not justified; approximately 90% of patients with ACS would be better off with intensive medical therapy. The few who could benefit can be identified by transcranial Doppler embolus detection or features of vulnerable plaque that can be imaged by 3-dimensional ultrasound, MRI or positron emission tomography/computed tomography; some of these methods are still in development.

Carotid artery stenting is a less invasive alternative to endarterectomy to treat symptomatic carotid stenosis. Clinical trials showed a higher periprocedural risk of nondisabling stroke with stenting, and a higher periprocedural risk of myocardial infarction, cranial nerve palsy, and access site hematoma with endarterectomy. The excess in procedure-related strokes with stenting is mainly seen in patients aged 70 and over. After the procedural period, stenting and endarterectomy are equally effective in preventing stroke and recurrent carotid stenosis in the medium to long term. The choice of stenting versus endarterectomy should take into account risks of both procedures in individual patients.

Of the ≈ 795,000 strokes in the United States annually, 185,000 are recurrent. A third to half of them occur while on antiplatelet therapy. Multiple reasons could explain breakthrough stroke while on antiplatelet therapy. Management of recurrent stroke requires a meticulous search for the cause and mechanism of stroke. At present, there is no indication for antiplatelet resistance testing in ischemic stroke, or adjusting medications based on its results. Recent trials have shown the effectiveness of dual antiplatelet therapy in the acute period after an ischemic event, but no benefit has been found with this regimen for long-term secondary prevention.

Patent foramen ovale (PFO) is common and only rarely related to stroke. The high PFO prevalence in healthy individuals makes for difficult decision making when a PFO is found in the setting of a cryptogenic stroke, because the PFO may be an incidental finding. Recent clinical trials of device-based PFO closure have had negative overall summary results; these trials have been limited by low recurrence rates. The optimal antithrombotic strategy for these patients is also unknown. Recent work has identified a risk score that estimates PFO-attributable fractions based on individual patient characteristics, although whether this score can help direct therapy is unclear.

Although screening for hypercoagulable states is commonly performed as part of the evaluation of first arterial ischemic stroke in young adults, available evidence does not support this as a routine practice, even in patients with cryptogenic stroke and a positive family history of early thrombotic events or in patients with a patent foramen ovale. Testing for antiphospholipid antibodies is a possible exception because persistent antibodies are associated with an increased risk of recurrent stroke. Despite the lack of supporting data, screening for hypercoagulable states in recurrent early-onset cryptogenic cerebral ischemia could be considered.

Primary angiitis of the central nervous system (PACNS) is a vasculitis of small arteries and veins of unknown cause restricted to the central nervous system (CNS), and controversy and disagreement exist over the means to establish the diagnosis. Cerebral arteriography, cerebrospinal fluid examination, and MRI singly or in combination do not have sufficiently demonstrated positive predictive value to establish the diagnosis. An alternative diagnosis is established at biopsy in 35% of cases. Histologic confirmation is required for the diagnosis of PACNS. Patients without histologic confirmation should not be included in case reports, case series, or reviews.

NEUROLOGIC CLINICS

RELATED INTEREST

Neuroimaging Clinics of North America, November 2013 (Vol. 23, No. 4)
Endovascular Management of Neurovascular Pathology in Adults and Children
Neeraj Chaudhary and Joseph J. Gemmete, *Editors*

NOW AVAILABLE FOR YOUR iPhone and iPad

Preface

Cerebrovascular Diseases: Controversies and Challenges

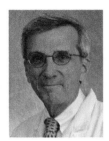

William J. Powers, MD
Editor

This issue of *Neurologic Clinics* is devoted to cerebrovascular disease. Over the past four decades, the field of cerebrovascular diseases has progressed from recommendations based on experience and opinion to guidelines based on data from multiple, well-executed, randomized clinical trials. Nevertheless, there remain areas of uncertainty and controversy for which current data available from clinical trials have failed to produce consensus within the community of stroke practitioners. For this issue, thirteen of these areas were selected, and experts in each area were asked to provide up-to-date articles defining the problem, reviewing pertinent data, describing the areas of controversy, and providing conclusions regarding efficacy based on the available evidence. The thirteen topics include treatments for acute ischemic stroke and intracerebral hemorrhage, prevention of subsequent stroke (in patients with symptomatic and asymptomatic carotid stenosis, cervical artery dissection, patent foramen ovale, unruptured arteriovenous malformations, and "aspirin failure"), and the appropriate use of diagnostic testing for intracerebral hemorrhage, hypercoagulability, and suspected primary angiitis of the central nervous system. I am deeply grateful to all the authors who devoted their time to writing such high-quality articles that I had very little to do and learned a lot.

I would also like to express my gratitude to Elsevier for providing me the opportunity to organize and edit this issue and to the editorial staff at *Neurologic Clinics* for their assistance in making it an easy task.

William J. Powers, MD
H. Houston Merritt Distinguished Professor and Chair
Department of Neurology
University of North Carolina at Chapel Hill
Room 2131, CB #7025, 170 Manning Drive
Chapel Hill, NC 27514, USA

E-mail address:
powersw@neurology.unc.edu

Neurol Clin 33 (2015) xiii
http://dx.doi.org/10.1016/j.ncl.2015.02.001
0733-8619/15/$ – see front matter © 2015 Published by Elsevier Inc.

neurologic.theclinics.com

Note on Levels of Clinical Efficacy

In this issue of *Neurologic Clinics*, authors were asked to provide an evidence-based evaluation of clinical efficacy of therapeutic interventions and diagnostic tests using the classification scheme in **Box 1**. Although heavily based on classification schemes used by the American Heart Association, the National Stroke Association, and the American Academy of Neurology, this new scheme was meant to address 2 perceived shortcomings in current schemes.[1–5] This scheme preserves the primacy of evidence of controlled trials over other evidence consistent with the National Stroke Association, American Academy of Neurology, and pre-2006 American Heart Association classifications.[1–3] More importantly, this scheme bases the clinical efficacy of diagnostic testing on the effect of the test in altering patient outcome, not just on accuracy or

---

Box 1
Levels of clinical efficacy

Clinical Efficacy of Therapeutic Interventions

Levels of evidence (modified from Johnston and colleagues[1])

Category T1: Based on evidence drawn from randomized, controlled trials (RCTs), or meta-analyses based on RCTs, with a clinically meaningful endpoint, that have narrow confidence intervals, a low risk for bias, and consistent results

Category T2: Based on evidence drawn from RCTs, or meta-analyses of such trials, with a clinically meaningful endpoint, that have wide confidence intervals, a higher risk for bias, or inconsistent results

Category T3: Based on evidence drawn from prospective observational studies, including cohort studies with concurrent controls and case-control studies that have a clinically meaningful endpoint

Category T4: Based on evidence drawn from other studies that have a clinically meaningful endpoint, including retrospective studies, descriptive studies, cross-sectional studies, case series, and reports. Prospective cohort studies using historical controls are included, together with expert medical opinion and general consensus. Results from RCTs that are based on biomarkers are also included in this category.

Levels of Clinical Efficacy (modified from Gronseth and French[2])

1. Established as beneficial (1-1), ineffective (1-0), or harmful (1-X) for changing meaningful clinical outcome for the given condition in the specified population (category T1 evidence or extensive consistent T3 evidence)

2. Probably beneficial (2-1), ineffective (2-0), or harmful (2-X) for changing meaningful clinical outcome for the given condition in the specified population (at least category T2 evidence or extensive consistent T3 evidence)

3. Possibly beneficial (3-1), ineffective (3-0), or harmful (3-X) for changing meaningful clinical outcome for the given condition in the specified population (category T3 or T4 evidence)

U. Unknown effectiveness: data inadequate or conflicting; given current knowledge, treatment is unproven/unknown

---

Neurol Clin 33 (2015) xv–xvii
http://dx.doi.org/10.1016/j.ncl.2015.02.002
0733-8619/15/$ – see front matter © 2015 Published by Elsevier Inc.
neurologic.theclinics.com

Clinical Efficacy of Diagnostic Tests

Levels of Evidence

Category D1A: Based on RCTs, or meta-analyses based on RCTs, with consistent results, narrow confidence intervals, and a low risk for bias in which patients are prospectively randomized to receive the diagnostic test or not and the outcome is a clinically meaningful endpoint

Category D1B: Based on RCTs, or meta-analyses based on RCTs, with inconsistent results, wide confidence intervals, or a higher risk for bias in which patients are prospectively randomized to receive the diagnostic test or not and the outcome is a clinically meaningful endpoint

Category D2A: Based on RCTs, or meta-analyses based on RCTs, with consistent results, narrow confidence intervals, and a low risk for bias in which the results of the diagnostic test are an eligibility criterion and the outcome is a clinically meaningful endpoint

Category D2B: Based on RCTs, or meta-analyses based on RCTs with inconsistent results, wide confidence intervals, or a higher risk for bias in which the results of the diagnostic test are an eligibility criterion and the outcome is a clinically meaningful endpoint

Category D3: Based on evidence drawn from prospective observational studies, including cohort studies with concurrent controls and case-control studies in which the results of the diagnostic test were used to guide therapy and the outcome is a clinically meaningful endpoint

Category D4: Based on evidence drawn from other studies that have a clinically meaningful endpoint in which the results of the diagnostic test are used to guide therapy, including retrospective studies, descriptive studies, cross-sectional studies, case series, and reports. Prospective cohort studies using historical controls are included, together with expert medical opinion and general consensus. Results from RCTs that are based on biomarkers also included in this category.

Levels of Clinical Efficacy (modified from Gronseth and French[2])

Established as beneficial (1-1), ineffective (1-0), or harmful (1-X) for changing meaningful clinical outcome for the given condition in the specified population when used to guide therapy (category D1A evidence)

1. Probably beneficial (2-1), ineffective (2-0), or harmful (2-X) for changing meaningful clinical outcome for the given condition in the specified population when used to guide therapy (at least category D1B or D2A evidence)

2. Possibly beneficial (3-1), ineffective (3-0), or harmful (3-X) for changing meaningful clinical outcome for the given condition in the specified population when used to guide therapy (at least category D2B, D3, or D4 evidence)

   U. Unknown effectiveness: Data inadequate or conflicting; given current knowledge, treatment is unproven/unknown

predictive value. This approach, based on work by Fineberg and colleagues, Fryback and Thornbury, and Kent and Larson, is lacking in some currently used criteria.[5-9]

William J. Powers, MD
Department of Neurology
University of North Carolina School of Medicine
Chapel Hill, NC, USA

E-mail address:
powersw@neurology.unc.edu

REFERENCES

1. Johnston SC, Nguyen-Huynh MN, Schwarz ME, et al. National Stroke Association guidelines for the management of transient ischemic attacks. Ann Neurol 2006;60: 301–13.
2. Gronseth G, French J. Practice parameters and technology assessments: what they are, what they are not, and why you should care. Neurology 2008;71:1639–43.
3. Adams H, Adams R, Del Zoppo G, et al. Guidelines for the early management of patients with ischemic stroke: 2005 guidelines update a scientific statement from the Stroke Council of the American Heart Association/American Stroke Association. Stroke 2005;36:916–23.
4. Sacco RL, Adams R, Albers G, et al. Guidelines for prevention of stroke in patients with ischemic stroke or transient ischemic attack: a statement for healthcare professionals from the American Heart Association/American Stroke Association Council on Stroke: co-sponsored by the Council on Cardiovascular Radiology and Intervention: the American Academy of Neurology affirms the value of this guideline. Stroke 2006;37:577–617.
5. Muayqil T, Gronseth G, Camicioli R. Evidence-based guideline: diagnostic accuracy of CSF 14-3-3 protein in sporadic Creutzfeldt-Jakob disease: report of the guideline development subcommittee of the American Academy of Neurology. Neurology 2012;79:1499–506.
6. Fineberg HV, Bauman R, Sosman M. Computerized cranial tomography. Effect on diagnostic and therapeutic plans. JAMA 1977;238:224–7.
7. Fryback DG, Thornbury JR. The efficacy of diagnostic imaging. Med Decis Making 1991;11:88–94.
8. Kent DL, Larson EB. Disease, level of impact, and quality of research methods. Three dimensions of clinical efficacy assessment applied to magnetic resonance imaging. Invest Radiol 1992;27:245–54.
9. Jauch EC, Saver JL, Adams HP Jr, et al. Guidelines for the early management of patients with acute ischemic stroke: a guideline for healthcare professionals from the American Heart Association/American Stroke Association. Stroke 2013;44: 870–947.

Diagnostic Evaluation for Nontraumatic Intracerebral Hemorrhage

Renan Domingues, MD[a,b], Costanza Rossi, MD, PhD[a],
Charlotte Cordonnier, MD, PhD[a,*]

KEYWORDS

- Intracerebral hemorrhage • Deep perforating vasculopathy
- Cerebral amyloid angiopathy • Diagnostic evaluation • MRI
- Digital subtraction angiography

KEY POINTS

- The incidence of intracerebral hemorrhage (ICH) ranges from 15 to 40 per 100,000 person-years. ICH is a devastating condition, with a 30-day mortality ranging from 35% to 52% with only 20% of survivors achieving full functional recovery at 6 months.
- Several different underlying vessel diseases may result in ICH. The aim of the diagnostic evaluation is not only to confirm the ICH diagnosis but also to establish the cause of the bleeding.
- Noncontrast computed tomography is highly sensitive for the detection of clinically relevant acute brain hemorrhage but the most useful tool for the etiologic evaluation of ICH is MRI. Besides being highly sensitive, MRI provides clues to the underlying vessel disease. Other neuroimaging techniques, such as CT angiography, magnetic resonance angiography and magnetic resonance venography, and digital subtraction angiography, can also be used to assess the intracranial vessels (arteries and veins).
- Diagnostic algorithms may vary according to the suspected underlying vessel disease.

INTRODUCTION

Intracerebral hemorrhage (ICH) is defined as a focal collection of blood within the brain parenchyma that may extend to other compartments of the brain (ventricular,

---

Disclosures: R. Domingues has no disclosures. C. Rossi was investigator in Brainsgate (Impact-24), Astra-Zeneca (SOCRATES), Pfizer (A9951024). No personal funding, all honoraria were paid to Adrinoid or Lille University Hospital. C. Cordonnier was investigator in Photothera (NEST3), Brainsgate (Impact-24), Astra-Zeneca (SOCRATES). She is principal investigator in France for Pfizer (A9951024). She received speaker fees from Bayer, BMS. No personal funding, all honoraria were paid to Adrinoid or Lille University Hospital.
^a Department of Neurology, University of Lille, UDSL, CHU Lille, Inserm U 1171, Lille 59000, France; ^b CAPES Foundation, Ministry of Education, Quadra 2, Bloco L, Lote 06, Edifício Capes - CEP: 70.040-020 - Brasilia-DF, Brazil
* Corresponding author. Department of Neurology, University of Lille, UDSL, CHU Lille, Inserm U 1171, Lille Cedex 59037, France.
E-mail address: charlotte.cordonnier@chru-lille.fr

0733-8619/15/$ – see front matter © 2015 Elsevier Inc. All rights reserved.

subarachnoid, or subdural spaces). It is a heterogeneous condition resulting from several distinct underlying vasculopathies. The overall incidence of ICH ranges from 15 to 40 per 100,000 person-years.[1,2] ICH accounts for 10% to 15% of all strokes, but this proportion may be higher in Asian and African populations.[2] Despite a significant improvement in the management of ischemic strokes, ICH treatment has not significantly evolved and this condition remains associated with a very high case fatality rate in the first month, ranging from 13% to 61% of patients, with a median of 40% across studies.[2] The poor prognosis of ICH may be partly caused by poor understanding of this heterogeneous condition.

The clinical and epidemiologic scenario of ICH has been changing in the last decades.[3,4] Despite an overall stable incidence of ICH, the incidence among people younger than 60 years has decreased, whereas in those older than 75 years it has increased in association with increasing premorbid use of antithrombotic drugs at this age. This trend may suggest that some bleeding-prone vasculopathies in the elderly are more likely to bleed when antithrombotic drugs are used, as illustrated by the rise in the incidence of lobar ICH in the elderly, in which cerebral amyloid angiopathy (CAA) may be strongly implicated.[4]

WHAT ARE THE CAUSES TO SEARCH FOR IN PATIENTS WITH INTRACEREBRAL HEMORRHAGE?

Importance of Intracerebral Hemorrhage Location to Tailor Diagnostic Work-Up

ICH location can be classified as deep, lobar, and infratentorial (involving the cerebellum and/or the brainstem). The anatomical distribution of the hemorrhage and its extension to other compartments (subarachnoid, subdural, intraventricular) may contribute to identify the underlying cause of the bleeding.

Deep locations represent about 45% of all ICH, whereas lobar locations account for 30% to 40%, cerebellar for approximately 10%, and brainstem for approximately 5%. These proportions are subject to bias because most estimates are based on hospital series in which referral is less often considered for moribund patients or for patients with mild deficits, and on population studies that contain such a small proportion of ICH that any subdivisions are subject to chance effect.[5,6] The pooled 1-year survival estimate in nine population-based studies was 45.4% to 59.1% after lobar ICH and 45.4% to 59.5% after deep ICH.[7]

Causes of Intracerebral Hemorrhage

The two most frequent causes of ICH are deep perforating vasculopathy and CAA.

Deep perforating vasculopathy

Deep perforating vasculopathy accounts for nearly 50% of ICH worldwide.[8] Chronic arterial hypertension is the most frequent risk factor associated with deep perforating vasculopathy.[5] Deep perforating vasculopathy results probably from a reactive hyperplasia and microscopic degenerative changes of vessel wall components leading to reduced vascular reactivity and enhanced vessel wall fragility.[9] Deep perforating vasculopathy usually occurs in lenticulostriate arteries originating from middle cerebral artery, in small thalamic arteries arising from the posterior communicating and posterior cerebral arteries, and perforating arteries that arise from the basilar artery. Given the absence of anatomic demonstration of perforating arteries in the cerebellum, the implication of deep perforating vasculopathy in cerebellar ICH remains controversial.

Cerebral amyloid angiopathy
CAA-related ICH preferentially affects cortical-subcortical (lobar) regions, less commonly the cerebellum and rarely deep or brainstem structures, reflecting the distribution of the underlying microangiopathy.[10] CAA results from the progressive deposition of amyloid-β peptide in the walls of small-to-medium sized leptomeningeal and cortical vessels, reducing the vessels compliance, resulting in a spectrum of hemorrhagic manifestations varying from cerebral microhemorrhages to symptomatic ICH. Other neuropathologic features are associated with CAA, such as cortical microinfarcts and white matter hyperintensities, probably reflecting reduced perfusion by CAA-affected arteries.[11] CAA-related ICH accounts for at least 5% to 20% of all spontaneous ICH.[12]

The Boston criteria (**Table 1**) were proposed to estimate the likelihood of CAA in ICH. The categories of probable and possible CAA were based on the pattern and number of hemorrhagic lesions on neuroimaging.[13] These criteria are widely used but a few limitations have to be highlighted.[14] In the original version, the authors only took into account patients with symptomatic lobar ICH, but did not consider other CAA clinical manifestations, such as cognitive decline or focal transient neurologic symptoms. Furthermore, the value of other MRI biomarkers of CAA, such as the presence of lobar cerebral microbleeds (CMB) and superficial siderosis (see neuroimaging findings), for improving diagnostic performance of the Boston criteria needs further study.

Many other conditions are implicated in ICH pathogenesis,[15] such as intracranial vascular malformations (IVM; arteriovenous malformation, arteriovenous fistulas, cerebral cavernous malformations), hemorrhagic transformation of an ischemic stroke,[16] coagulopathies, drug abuse, brain tumor or metastases,[17] cerebral venous thrombosis,[18] and reversible cerebral vasoconstriction syndrome.[19]

DIAGNOSTIC WORK-UP
Clinical Presentation

The clinical presentation of ICH usually includes nonspecific symptoms (eg, headache and/or decreased consciousness), and focal symptoms that change according to the anatomic distribution of the ICH. The symptoms installation may be abrupt or gradual. Progressive clinical deterioration is a common presentation of ICH. Early hemorrhage growth is the most common identifiable factor associated with clinical deterioration and it is frequent: 38% of patients with ICH suffer from more than a 33% growth in the volume of parenchymal hemorrhage during the first 20 hours after the baseline computed tomography (CT) following admission. Most of the ongoing bleeding occurs within the first 3 to 4 hours after hemorrhage onset.[20] These data highlight the urgent need to consider ICH as a vital emergency as clinicians do with ischemic stroke or myocardial infarct.

Main Clinical Symptoms

Headache
In the first 12 hours, headaches are present in nearly one-third of patients admitted for ICH. The headaches are more frequent in ICH than in ischemic stroke (36% vs 16%) but headache characteristics are not reliable to distinguish these two types of stroke.[21] Patients with small or deep hemorrhage rarely have headache. Lobar ICH, cerebellar ICH, and the presence of meningeal signs are significantly associated with headache at onset of ICH.[22]

Nausea and vomiting
Nausea and vomiting are reported in 51% of patients with ICH.[23] In the posterior fossa, vomiting is a frequent symptom of ICH because of the dysfunction of vestibular

Table 1
Boston criteria for diagnosis of CAA in patients suffering from a lobar ICH

	Classic Boston Criteria	Modified Boston Criteria
Definite CAA	Full postmortem examination demonstrating • Lobar, cortical, or corticosubcortical hemorrhage[a] • Severe CAA with vasculopathy • Absence of other diagnostic lesion[b]	No modification compared with the classic Boston criteria
Probable CAA with supporting pathology	Clinical data and pathologic tissue (evacuated hematoma or cortical biopsy) demonstrating • Lobar, cortical, or corticosubcortical hemorrhage[a] • Some degree of CAA in specimen • Absence of other diagnostic lesion[b]	No modification compared with the classic Boston criteria
Probable CAA	Clinical data and MRI or CT demonstrating • Multiple hemorrhages[a] restricted to lobar, cortical, or corticosubcortical regions (cerebellar hemorrhage allowed) • Age ≥55 y • Absence of other cause of hemorrhage[b]	Clinical data and MRI or CT demonstrating • Multiple hemorrhages[a] restricted to lobar, cortical, or corticosubcortical regions (cerebellar hemorrhage allowed) or • Single lobar, cortical, or corticosubcortical hemorrhage and focal[c] or disseminated[d] superficial siderosis • Age ≥55 y • Absence of other cause of hemorrhage or superficial siderosis[b]
Possible CAA	Clinical data and MRI or CT demonstrating • Single lobar, cortical, or corticosubcortical hemorrhage[a] • Age ≥55 y • Absence of other cause of hemorrhage[b]	Clinical data and MRI or CT demonstrating • Single lobar, cortical, or corticosubcortical hemorrhage[a] and focal[c] or disseminated[d] superficial siderosis • Age ≥55 y • Absence of other cause of hemorrhage or superficial siderosis[b]

Abbreviations: CAA, cerebral amyloid angiopathy; CT, computed tomography; ICH, intracerebral hemorrhage.

[a] The term "hemorrhage" referred, in the pathologic validation, to lobar ICH. However, some authors suggest that multiple lobar cerebral microbleeds, without lobar ICH, may be considered as probable CAA.

[b] Other causes of ICH that question the diagnosis of CAA are excessive warfarin dose (INR>3.0; INR≤3 or other nonspecific laboratory abnormalities are permitted for diagnosis of possible CAA), antecedent of head trauma or ischemic stroke, hemorrhagic transformation of an ischemic stroke, arteriovenous malformation, central nervous system tumor or vasculitis, blood dyscrasia or coagulopathy.

[c] Siderosis restricted to three or fewer sulci.

[d] Siderosis affecting at least four sulci.

Adapted from Linn J, Halpin A, Demaerel P, et al. Prevalence of superficial siderosis in patients with cerebral amyloid angiopathy. Neurology 2010;74:1346–50.

structures or hemorrhage in the fourth ventricle. Vomiting is frequently present also in supratentorial hemorrhages probably because of increased intracranial pressure or ventricular extension.[24]

Seizures
The reported incidence of post-ICH seizures depends on study design, diagnostic criteria, duration of follow-up, and the population studied. It ranges from 2.8%[25] to 22.6%.[26] This great discrepancy reflects substantial methodologic differences among the studies. Most of the studies used a clinical definition for the seizures, but the studies using continuous electroencephalogram monitoring reported higher incidence of electrical seizures.[27] In a prospective series of 761 patients with ICH, 4.2% presented seizures in the first 24 hours. The seizures were partial simple in 62.5% and generalized in 28.1%. Lobar location was the most powerful predictor of seizures (odds ratio, 4.05; 95% confidence interval, 3.45–4.65).[28]

In a recent prospective study, early seizures (within 7 days after ICH) occurred in 14% of patients with ICH. Cortical involvement of ICH was the only factor associated with early seizures, half of which occurred at onset. Factors associated with onset seizures were previous ICH, cortical involvement, younger age, and severity of the neurologic deficit at admission.[29]

Decreased level of consciousness
In a large stroke data bank, only 28% of patients with ICH had normal level of consciousness, 31% had Glasgow Coma Scale between 9 and 14, 18% had Glasgow Coma Scale between 6 and 8, and 23% had Glasgow Coma Scale between 3 and 5.[30] Electroencephalogram monitoring is very helpful in patients with reduced level of consciousness to exclude nonconvulsive epileptic seizures that are frequently underdiagnosed in patients with ICH.[31]

Diagnostic Scales
Some clinical scales, such as Guy's Hospital Stroke Score and Siriraj Stroke Score, were proposed for the distinction between ischemic and hemorrhagic stroke. They take into account some clinical features more commonly found in hemorrhagic than in ischemic stroke, such as loss of consciousness, headache at the onset, vomiting, and neck stiffness.[32,33] However, validation studies showed that none of them are reliable for diagnosis of ICH, emphasizing the need for routine neuroimaging evaluation.[34]

Prognostic Scales
Several clinical grading scales for ICH have been used to predict vital or functional outcome at the time of presentation.[35–37] Among these, the ICH Score is the most commonly used (**Table 2**). The ICH Score ranges from 0 (excellent prognosis) to 6 (high probability of death).[35] This score correlates well with 30-day mortality and 1-year functional outcome.[38] Although ICH Score and other clinical grading scales may be useful for prognostic evaluation, other factors, including the underlying cause of the ICH, also influence the ICH prognosis. For example, patients with ICH related to an arteriovenous malformation had better outcomes than patients with other causes of ICH, independently of other known predictors of outcome.[39]

Do-not-resuscitate (DNR) orders are relatively common in patients with ICH, especially among those with expected poor prognosis. In a recent study, DNR orders were issued in 35% out of 1013 patients with ICH. Advanced age, more severe stroke, and early deterioration were associated with higher probability of DNR orders. Patients with DNR orders received less active care.[40] Use of ICH predictive models without

Table 2 Determination of ICH score	
Component	**ICH Score Points**
GCS score	
3–4	2
5–12	1
13–15	0
ICH volume in cm³	
≥30	1
<30	0
IVH	
Yes	1
No	0
Infratentorial origin of ICH	
Yes	1
No	0
Age, y	
≥80	1
<80	0
Total ICH score	0–6

Abbreviations: GCS, Glasgow coma score; ICH, intracerebral hemorrhage; IVH, intraventricular hemorrhage.

From Hemphill JC III, Bonovich DC, Besmertis L, et al. The ICH score: a simple, reliable grading scale for intracerebral hemorrhage. Stroke 2001;32:891–7; with permission.

considering the impact of early DNR orders may lead to inaccurate estimates of mortality risk for individual patients.[41]

Clinical Clues

The medical history may provide useful information for elucidating the cause of ICH:

- Age: younger age may suggest the diagnosis of an IVM, whereas old age is more often associated with deep perforating vasculopathy and CAA
- A family history of ICH may suggest cerebral cavernous malformations and other IVMs, and rare genetic familial forms of CAA
- Previous epileptic seizures or previous ICH in the same territory should raise suspicion about an IVM or a tumor
- Previous history of cognitive decline and transient focal neurologic symptoms ("amyloid spells") may suggest CAA
- If the patient is known to have had cancer, hemorrhage into a brain metastasis should be excluded
- Illicit drugs use should be screened, especially cocaine and amphetamines among young patients with ICH
- Pregnancy and puerperium are potentially associated with eclampsia, choriocarcinoma, and cerebral venous thrombosis

Clinical examination may rarely provide etiologic clues. Diffuse ecchymoses or bleeding may suggest coagulopathy. A cardiac murmur may suggest septic embolism. Cutaneous tumors may raise suspicion of metastasis of melanoma. Hypertensive retinopathy seen at fundoscopic examination may be suggestive of a deep perforating vasculopathy.

Biologic Tests

Biologic tests rarely detect the cause of ICH but they can provide indirect information that can contribute to the diagnostic evaluation (eg, an inflammatory condition in a patient with angiitis, coagulation tests abnormalities, liver enzyme changes in alcoholism). Biologic evaluation should include the following tests:

- Blood cell counts
- Prothrombin time, international normalized ratio, partial thromboplastin time
- C-reactive protein, fibrinogen levels, blood cultures (in cases of suspected infection)
- Liver enzymes
- Creatinine and blood urea nitrogen levels
- Screening for prothrombotic conditions in cases of cerebral venous thrombosis when indicated. The most common trombophilic disorders are factor V Leyden mutation, prothrombin G20210A mutation, protein C deficiency, protein S deficiency, antithrombin III deficiency, elevated factor VIII, antiphospholipid antibody syndrome, hyperhomocysteinemia, and activated protein C resistance. A hypercoagulable state should be investigated in patients with unexplained cerebral venous thrombosis.[42]
- Screening for illicit drugs: cocaine metabolites can be screened in urine within 48 hours of admission.[43,44] Recently, other fluids, such as oral fluid, hair, and sweat, have been used to detect cocaine and its metabolites.[45]

The association between ICH and the use of amphetamines, cocaine (and its freebase form crack-cocaine), and ecstasy has been reported with increasingly frequency.[46,47] Cocaine-associated ICH is more frequent in males with a high proportion of subcortical ICH.[43] Poorer outcome was shown in cocaine-associated ICH.[42]

Neuroimaging Findings

Noncontrast computerized tomography

Noncontrast CT is the most rapid and readily available tool for the diagnosis of ICH, being the most commonly used neuroimaging tool in emergency departments. ICH appears as a hyperdense lesion within minutes after the onset of symptoms but noncontrast CT has decreased sensitivity 1 week after ICH onset because the lesion becomes isodense with respect to the brain parenchyma. Noncontrast CT allows the identification of anatomic distribution of the hematoma, extension to ventricular system, and an estimation of hematoma volume.[48]

Computed tomography angiography

CT angiography (CTA) has been used as a tool to predict hemorrhage enlargement by revealing a spot sign. Spot sign was first described in 1999 and is defined as a contrast extravasation within the hematoma. The supposed cause is continued bleeding from ruptured vessels, but the precise mechanism is still poorly understood.[49] One prospective study suggested that the spot sign may have value to predict ICH enlargement (positive predictive value of 73%, negative predictive value of 84%, sensitivity of 63%, and specificity of 90%). In this study, patients with ICH with a spot sign had a worse prognosis than patients without a spot sign.[50] CTA has also shown promising results for the detection of underlying vasculopathy in young patients with lobar ICH,[51] but further studies are still needed to assess CTA diagnostic accuracy for all patients with ICH.

MRI

The accuracy of MRI to detect acute symptomatic ICH is equivalent to CT. Moreover, MRI is more sensitive than CT to detect chronic hemorrhage.[52] The imaging characteristics of ICH vary with time (**Fig. 1**). In the acute phase, gradient echo T2*-weighted MRI is the most sensitive sequence, whereas the other MRI sequences may give indirect clues for etiologic diagnosis.

MRI radiologic markers, such as white matter hyperintensities of presumed vascular origin, lacunes, deep CMB, and brain atrophy, are suggestive of deep perforating vasculopathy (**Fig. 2**).[53]

Several MRI findings point toward the diagnosis of CAA (**Fig. 3**). Strictly lobar CMBs have been associated with CAA in clinical and genetic studies.[54,55] Superficial siderosis is probably linked to repeated bleeding episodes in the subarachnoid or subpial space and may be responsible for transient focal neurologic symptoms and seizures.[56] White matter hyperintensities may occur in CAA and probably result from the accumulation of silent ischemic lesions as a consequence of CAA-associated cerebral small-vessel disease and may be a predictor of disease burden.[57] Moreover, a more posterior distribution of white matter hyperintensities was recently found to be an independent predictor of CAA diagnosis and may represent an additional marker of

	Phase of blood	T1	T2	Flair	T2* GRE
Hyperacute	Oxyhemoglobin				
Acute (12-48h)	Deoxyhemoglobin				
Early subacute (2-7d)	Methemoglobin intracellular				
Late subacute (8d-1m)	Methemoglobin extracellular				
Chronic (>1m)	Hemosiderin and ferritin				

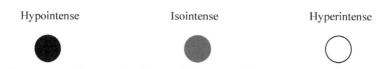

Hypointense   Isointense   Hyperintense

Fig. 1. Appearance of intracerebral hemorrhage on MRI by stage. GRE, gradient echo. (*Data from* Kidwell CS, Chalela JA, Saver JL, et al. Comparison of MRI and CT for detection of acute intracerebral hemorrhage. JAMA 2004;292:1823–30; and Wijman CA, Venkatasubramanian C, Bruins S, et al. Utility of early MRI diagnosis and management of acute spontaneous intracerebral haemorrhage. Cerebrovasc Dis 2010;30:456–63.)

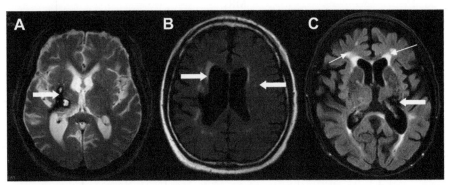

Fig. 2. Deep perforating vasculopathy MRI findings. (*A*) Axial slice, T2* gradient echo, showing right thalamic hemorrhage (*arrow*). (*B*) Axial slice, FLAIR sequence of patient from A, showing a characteristic feature of deep perforating vasculopathy in its occlusive expression: periventricular white matter lesions (*arrows*). (*C*) Axial slice, FLAIR sequence, showing a chronic left thalamic hemorrhage (*thick arrow*) and extensive white matter disease involving periventricular regions, resulting from deep perforating vasculopathy in its occlusive expression (*thin arrows*).

CAA.[58] Silent microinfarcts have also been associated with CAA. They are correlated with white matter changes and CMB, suggesting that they result from an occlusive small-vessel arteriopathy.[59] Enlarged or dilated white-matter perivascular spaces, presumed to be caused by the accumulation of interstitial fluid, have been linked to the presence and severity of cerebral small-vessel disease. Severe centrum semiovale enlarged perivascular spaces seem to be associated with CAA, whereas basal ganglia enlarged perivascular space seems to be associated with deep perforating vasculopathy.[60,61]

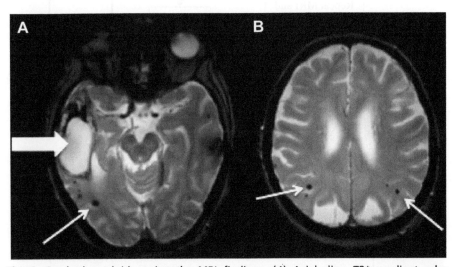

Fig. 3. Cerebral amyloid angiopathy MRI findings. (*A*) Axial slice, T2* gradient echo, showing a right lobar temporal hemorrhage (*thick arrow*) and lobar cerebral microbleeds (*thin arrow*). (*B*) Axial slice, T2* gradient echo, showing right and left lobar cerebral microbleeds (*arrows*).

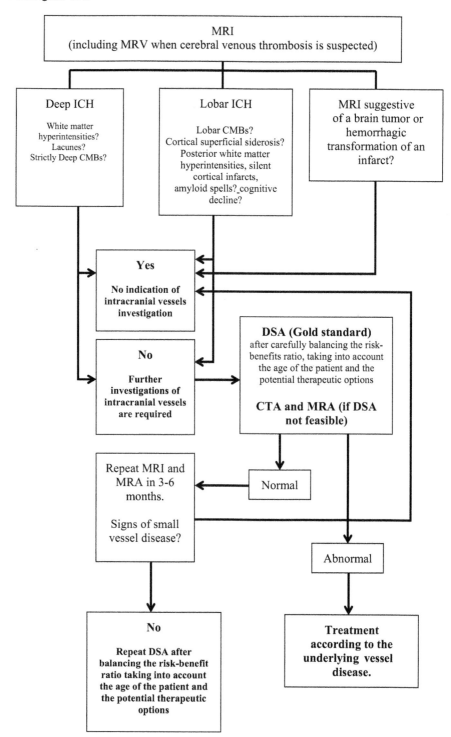

Fig. 4. ICH diagnostic decision tree. CMB, cerebral microbleeds; CTA, computed tomography angiography; DSA, digital subtraction angiography; ICH, intracerebral hemorrhage; MRA, magnetic resonance angiography; MRV, magnetic resonance venography.

Intracranial vessels evaluation
Magnetic resonance angiography and magnetic resonance venography, CTA and CT venography, and conventional digital subtraction angiography can be used in cases in which a vascular malformation or a cerebral venous thrombosis is suspected. Magnetic resonance angiography and magnetic resonance venography and CTA and CT venography constitute alternative methods to conventional digital subtraction angiography to detect IVMs and showed promising results in small studies.[62,63] However, conventional digital subtraction angiography remains the gold standard to disclose underlying vascular malformations in patients with ICH. This option should be discussed in all patients with ICH without any obvious cause.

Recommendations
Evidence-based recommendations are lacking for what concerns the type and timing of the neuroradiologic investigations.[64] The American Heart Association/American Stroke Association recommended[65] rapid neuroimaging with CT or MRI to distinguish ischemic stroke from ICH (Level A of evidence); and CTA or contrast-enhanced CT may be considered to help identify patients at risk for hematoma expansion (Level B of evidence) and vessel examination can be useful to screen for underlying structural lesions, including vascular malformations and tumors when there is a clinical or radiologic suspicion (Level B of evidence).

If the clinical condition of the patient allows, MRI is the best option in the setting of ICH. In addition to establishing the diagnosis of ICH, MRI may provide information that contributes to the etiologic diagnosis of ICH.[66,67] If the etiologic diagnosis was not firmly established in the acute phase, vessel examination should be repeated 3 to 6 months after ICH onset.[68] A decision tree, based on clinical experience rather than on evidence-based data, is proposed in **Fig. 4**.

SUMMARY

ICH remains a devastating disorder. The ICH classification into primary versus secondary should be replaced by an approach where the priority is rapid ICH diagnosis and elucidation of the underlying vessel disease. This paradigm might contribute to the development of new treatment strategies and the prevention of recurrent events.

REFERENCES

1. Feigin VL, Forouzanfar MH, Krishnamurthi R, et al. Global and regional burden of stroke during 1990–2010: findings from the Global Burden of Disease Study 2010. Lancet 2014;383:245–54.
2. van Asch CJ, Luitse MJ, Rinkel GJ, et al. Incidence, case fatality, and functional outcome of intracerebral haemorrhage over time, according to age, sex, and ethnic origin: a systematic review and meta-analysis. Lancet Neurol 2010;9: 167–76.
3. Lovelock CE, Molyneux AJ, Rothwell PM, et al. Change in incidence and aetiology of intracerebral haemorrhage in Oxfordshire, UK, between 1981 and 2006: a population-based study. Lancet Neurol 2007;6:487–93.
4. Béjot Y, Cordonnier C, Durier J, et al. Intracerebral haemorrhage profiles are changing: results from the Dijon population-based study. Brain 2013;136:658–64.
5. Sacco RL, Kasner SE, Broderick JP, et al. An updated definition of stroke for the 21st century: a statement for healthcare professionals from the American Heart Association/American Stroke Association. Stroke 2013;44:2064–89.
6. Warlow C, Sudlow C, Dennis M, et al. Stroke. Lancet 2003;362:1211–24.

7. Poon MT, Fonville AF, Al-Shahi Salman R. Long-term prognosis after intracerebral haemorrhage: systematic review and meta-analysis. J Neurol Neurosurg Psychiatr 2014;85:660–7.

8. Smith SD, Eskey CJ. Hemorrhagic stroke. Radiol Clin North Am 2011;49:27–45.

9. Fisher CM. Pathological observations in hypertensive cerebral hemorrhage. J Neuropathol Exp Neurol 1971;30:536–50.

10. Charidimou A, Gang Q, Werring DJ. Sporadic cerebral amyloid angiopathy revisited: recent insights into pathophysiology and clinical spectrum. J Neurol Neurosurg Psychiatr 2012;83:124–37.

11. Fisher M, French S, Ji P, et al. Cerebral microbleeds in the elderly: a pathological analysis. Stroke 2010;41:2782–5.

12. Maia LF, Mackenzie IR, Feldman HH. Clinical phenotypes of cerebral amyloid angiopathy. J Neurol Sci 2007;257:23–30.

13. Knudsen KA, Rosand J, Karluk D, et al. Clinical diagnosis of cerebral amyloid angiopathy: validation of the Boston criteria. Neurology 2001;56:537–9.

14. Samarasekera N, Smith C, Al-Shahi Salman R. The association between cerebral amyloid angiopathy and intracerebral haemorrhage: systematic review and meta-analysis. J Neurol Neurosurg Psychiatr 2012;83:275–81.

15. Al-Shahi Salman R, Labovitz DL, Stapf C. Spontaneous intracerebral haemorrhage. BMJ 2009;339:b2586.

16. Álvarez-Sabín J, Maisterra O, Santamarina E, et al. Factors influencing haemorrhagic transformation in ischaemic stroke. Lancet Neurol 2013;12:689–705.

17. Licata B, Turazzi S. Bleeding cerebral neoplasms with symptomatic hematoma. J Neurol Sci 2003;47:201–10.

18. Stam J. Thrombosis of the cerebral veins and sinuses. N Engl J Med 2005;352:1791–8.

19. Ducros A. Reversible cerebral vasoconstriction syndrome. Lancet Neurol 2012; 11:906–17.

20. Brott T, Broderick J, Kothari R, et al. Early hemorrhage growth in patients with intracerebral hemorrhage. Stroke 1997;28:1–5.

21. Kumral E, Bogousslavsky J, Van Melle G, et al. Headache at stroke onset: the Lausanne stroke registry. J Neurol Neurosurg Psychiatr 1995;58:490–2.

22. Melo TP, Pinto AN, Ferro JM. Headache in intracerebral hematomas. Neurology 1996;47:494–500.

23. Mohr JP, Caplan LR, Melski JW, et al. The Harvard cooperative stroke registry: a prospective registry. Neurology 1978;28:754–62.

24. Broderick JP, Adams HP Jr, Barsan W, et al. Guidelines for the management of spontaneous intracerebral hemorrhage: a statement for healthcare professionals from a special writing group of the Stroke Council, American Heart Association. Stroke 1999;30:905–15.

25. Sung CY, Chu NS. Epileptic seizures in intracerebral haemorrhage. J Neurol Neurosurg Psychiatr 1989;52:1273–6.

26. Szaflarski JP, Rackley AY, Kleindorfer DO, et al. Incidence of seizures in the acute phase of stroke: a population-based study. Epilepsia 2008;49:974–81.

27. Claassen J, Jetté N, Chum F, et al. Electrographic seizures and periodic discharges after intracerebral hemorrhage. Neurology 2007;69:1356–65.

28. Passero S, Rocchi R, Rossi S, et al. Seizures after spontaneous supratentorial intracerebral hemorrhage. Epilepsia 2002;43:1175–80.

29. De Herdt V, Dumont F, Hénon H, et al. Early seizures in intracerebral hemorrhage: incidence, associated factors, and outcome. Neurology 2011;77:1794–800.

30. Foulkes MA, Wolf PA, Price TR, et al. The stroke data bank: design, methods, and baseline characteristics. Stroke 1988;19:547–54.

31. Claassen J, Mayer SA, Kowalski RG, et al. Detection of electrographic seizures with continuous EEG monitoring in critically ill patients. Neurology 2004;62: 1743–8.
32. Allen CM. Clinical diagnosis of the acute stroke syndrome. Q J Med 1983;52: 515–23.
33. Poungvarin N, Viriyavejakul A, Komontri C. Siriraj stroke score and validation study to distinguish supratentorial intracerebral haemorrhage from infarction. BMJ 1991;302:1565–7.
34. Weir CJ, Murray GD, Adams FG, et al. Poor accuracy of stroke scoring systems for differential clinical diagnosis of intracranial haemorrhage and infarction. Lancet 1994;344:999–1002.
35. Hemphill JC III, Bonovich DC, Besmertis L, et al. The ICH score: a simple, reliable grading scale for intracerebral hemorrhage. Stroke 2001;32:891–7.
36. Cheung RT, Zou LY. Use of the original, modified, or new intracerebral hemorrhage score to predict mortality and morbidity after intracerebral hemorrhage. Stroke 2003;34:1717–22.
37. Rost NS, Smith EE, Chang Y, et al. Prediction of functional outcome in patients with primary intracerebral hemorrhage: the FUNC score. Stroke 2008;39:2304–9.
38. Hemphill JC III, Farrant M, Neill TA Jr. Prospective validation of the ICH Score for 12-month functional outcome. Neurology 2009;73:1088–94.
39. van Beijnum J, Lovelock CE, Cordonnier C, et al. Outcome after spontaneous and arteriovenous malformation-related intracerebral haemorrhage: population-based studies. Brain 2009;132:537–43.
40. Silvennoinen K, Meretoja A, Strbian D, et al. Do-not-resuscitate (DNR) orders in patients with intracerebral hemorrhage. Int J Stroke 2014;9:53–8.
41. Zahuranec DB, Morgenstern LB, Sánchez BN, et al. Do-not-resuscitate orders and predictive models after intracerebral hemorrhage. Neurology 2010;75: 626–33.
42. White RH, Gosselin RG. Testing for theombophilia: pitfalls, limitations, and marginal impact on treatment duration recommendations. Mt Sinai J Med 2009;76: 303–13.
43. Bajwa AA, Silliman S, Cury JD, et al. Characteristics and outcomes of cocaine-related spontaneous intracerebral hemorrhages. ISRN Neurol 2013;2013:124390.
44. Martin-Schild S, Albright KC, Hallevi H, et al. Intracerebral hemorrhage in cocaine users. Stroke 2010;41:680–4.
45. Bortolotti F, Gottardo R, Pascali J, et al. Toxicokinetics of cocaine and metabolites: the forensic toxicological approach. Curr Med Chem 2012;19:5658–63.
46. McEvoy AW, Kitchen ND, Thomas DG. Lesson of the week: intracerebral haemorrhage in young adults: the emerging importance of drug misuse. BMJ 2000;320: 1322–4.
47. Gee P, Tallon C, Long N, et al. Use of recreational drug 1,3 dimethylamylamine (DMAA) associated with cerebral hemorrhage. Ann Emerg Med 2012;60:431–4.
48. Caceres JA, Goldstein JN. Intracranial hemorrhage. Emerg Med Clin North Am 2012;30:771–94.
49. Brouwers HB, Goldstein JN, Romero JM, et al. Clinical applications of the computed tomography angiography spot sign in acute intracerebral hemorrhage: a review. Stroke 2012;43:3427–32.
50. Demchuk AM, Dowlatshahi D, Rodriguez-Luna D, et al. Prediction of haematoma growth and outcome in patients with intracerebral haemorrhage using the CT angiography spot sign (PREDICT): a prospective observational study. Lancet Neurol 2012;11:307–14.

51. Wong GK, Siu DY, Abrigo JM, et al. Computed tomographic angiography and venography for young or nonhypertensive patients with acute spontaneous intracerebral hemorrhage. Stroke 2011;42:211–3.
52. Kidwell CS, Chalela JA, Saver JL, et al. Comparison of MRI and CT for detection of acute intracerebral hemorrhage. JAMA 2004;292:1823–30.
53. Wardlaw JM, Smith C, Dichgans M. Mechanisms of sporadic cerebral small vessel disease: insights from neuroimaging. Lancet Neurol 2013;12:483–97.
54. Charidimou A, Werring DJ. Cerebral microbleeds as a predictor of macrobleeds: what is the evidence? Int J Stroke 2014;9:457–9.
55. O'Donnell HC, Rosand J, Knudsen KA, et al. Apolipoprotein E genotype and the risk of recurrent lobar intracerebral hemorrhage. N Engl J Med 2000;342:240–5.
56. Linn J, Herms J, Dichgans M, et al. Subarachnoid hemosiderosis and superficial cortical hemosiderosis in cerebral amyloid angiopathy. AJNR Am J Neuroradiol 2008;29:184–6.
57. Chen YW, Gurol ME, Rosand J, et al. Progression of white matter lesions and hemorrhages in cerebral amyloid angiopathy. Neurology 2006;67:83–7.
58. Thanprasertsuk S, Martinez-Ramirez S, Pontes-Neto OM, et al. Posterior white matter disease distribution as a predictor of amyloid angiopathy. Neurology 2014;83:794–800.
59. Gregoire SM, Charidimou A, Gadapa N, et al. Acute ischaemic brain lesions in intracerebral haemorrhage: multicentre cross-sectional magnetic resonance imaging study. Brain 2011;134:2376–86.
60. Charidimou A, Meegahage R, Fox Z, et al. Enlarged perivascular spaces as a marker of underlying arteriopathy in intracerebral haemorrhage: a multicentre MRI cohort study. J Neurol Neurosurg Psychiatr 2013;84:624–9.
61. Charidimou A, Jäger RH, Peeters A, et al. White matter perivascular spaces are related to cortical superficial siderosis in cerebral amyloid angiopathy. Stroke 2014;45(10):2930–5.
62. Evans AL, Coley SC, Wilkinson ID, et al. First-line investigation of acute intracerebral hemorrhage using dynamic magnetic resonance angiography. Acta Radiol 2005;46:625–30.
63. Hadizadeh DR, Kukuk GM, Steck DT, et al. Noninvasive evaluation of cerebral arteriovenous malformations by 4D-MRA for preoperative planning and postoperative follow-up in 56 patients: comparison with DSA and intraoperative findings. AJNR Am J Neuroradiol 2012;33:1095–101.
64. Cordonnier C, Klijn CJ, vna Beijnum J, et al. Radiological investigation of spontaneous intracerebral hemorrahage: systemic review and trinational survey. Stroke 2010;41:685–90.
65. Morgenstern LB, Hemphill JC III, Anderson C, et al. Guidelines for the management of spontaneous intracerebral hemorrhage: a guideline for healthcare professionals from the American Heart Association/American Stroke Association. Stroke 2010;41:2108–29.
66. Wijman CA, Venkatasubramanian C, Bruins S, et al. Utility of early MRI diagnosis and management of acute spontaneous intracerebral haemorrhage. Cerebrovasc Dis 2010;30:456–63.
67. Macellari F, Paciaroni M, Agnelli G, et al. Neuroimaging in intracerebral haemorrhage. Stroke 2014;45:903–8.
68. Hino A, Fujimoto M, Yamaki T, et al. Value of repeat angiography in patients with spontaneous subcortical hemorrhage. Stroke 1998;29:2517–21.

Antiplatelet and Anticoagulant Therapy After Intracerebral Hemorrhage

Allyson Zazulia, MD

KEYWORDS

- Intracerebral hemorrhage • Anticoagulation • Antiplatelet therapy • Atrial fibrillation
- Prosthetic heart valve • Venous thromboembolism

KEY POINTS

- Warfarin use is associated with an increased risk of hematoma expansion and poor outcome after intracerebral hemorrhage (ICH).
- The novel oral anticoagulants have a lower risk of hemorrhage than warfarin.
- Decisions about whether to resume antithrombotic therapy after ICH require individual assessment of the risk of thromboembolism versus risk of recurrent ICH.
- The risk of ICH recurrence is approximately 2% to 4% per year, with twofold higher rates reported for those with lobar ICH.
- Low-dose subcutaneous unfractionated and low molecular weight heparins are likely safe for use in venous thromboembolism prophylaxis in ICH after documentation of cessation of bleeding.
- Restarting anticoagulant therapy should be reserved for those patients who are at highest risk of thromboembolic events.
- In those who will resume oral anticoagulation, timing of when to restart is controversial; however, resumption at the end of the first week is typically reasonable; substituting a novel oral anticoagulant for warfarin is an attractive, although unproven, option for patients with atrial fibrillation or venous thromboembolism.
- Antiplatelet therapy is relatively safe after ICH; however, no antiplatelet therapy may be favored after lobar ICH.

ORAL ANTICOAGULANTS AND INTRACEREBRAL HEMORRHAGE
Background

Intracranial hemorrhage is one of the most feared complications of oral anticoagulant (OAC) therapy. The incidence of warfarin-associated intracerebral hemorrhage (ICH),

Financial Disclosures and Conflicts of Interest: None.
Department of Neurology, Washington University School of Medicine, 660 South Euclid Avenue, Campus Box 8111, St Louis, MO 63110, USA
E-mail address: zazuliaa@neuro.wustl.edu

0733-8619/15/$ – see front matter © 2015 Elsevier Inc. All rights reserved.

which comprises most warfarin-associated intracranial hemorrhages in stroke-prone patients, is approximately 1% per year, a rate that is 7 to 10 times higher than in stroke-prone patients not taking warfarin.[1] ICH accounts for approximately 90% of the deaths and most of the permanent disability in patients with warfarin-associated bleeding.[2] Compared with spontaneous ICH in nonanticoagulated patients, warfarin-associated hemorrhages tend to be larger regardless of whether the international normalized ratio (INR) is therapeutic or supratherapeutic, have a greater risk of hematoma enlargement, and have a higher mortality rate.[1]

The most consistently reported risk factors for warfarin-related ICH include advancing age (especially older than 75 years), Asian or black race, hypertension, history of cerebrovascular disease, presence of a prosthetic heart valve, and concomitant use of an antiplatelet agent.[3–5] Pharmacogenetic factors affect hemorrhage risk among warfarin users, with patients harboring the apolipoprotein ε2 or ε4 genotype, the cytochrome P450 CYP2C9*2 or *3 genotype, or the platelet glycoprotein IIb/IIIa A1A1 genotype having an increased risk. Also at increased risk are those with imaging evidence of cerebral microbleeds or leukoaraiosis.[6]

The risk of ICH doubles with each 0.5 increase in INR above the therapeutic range.[7] Most cases of warfarin-associated ICH occur when the INR is within a therapeutic range,[8] though, reflecting that most warfarin-treated patients are more commonly within this range than outside it.

Although definitive data are lacking, the most likely mechanism by which OAC use causes ICH is that it unmasks subclinical bleeding that occurs when vessels are damaged by aging, hypertension, microvasculopathy, or cerebrovascular disease (ie, it increases the likelihood that bleeding from spontaneously occurring arteriolar ruptures will not be stopped by normal hemostatic mechanisms). There is no pathogenetic rationale or data to support that OAC use promotes vascular injury, induces vessel rupture, or interferes with vessel repair.[9]

ICH occurring in the setting of warfarin use is associated with worse clinical outcome than spontaneous ICH, primarily based on 3 factors: (1) patients with warfarin-associated ICH tend to be older, (2) warfarin use is associated with larger baseline hemorrhages, and (3) warfarin use leads to a higher rate of hematoma enlargement. Hematoma enlargement occurs in more than one-third of patients with primary ICH, nearly always within 3 to 4 hours of onset, and increases the likelihood of neurologic deterioration and poor outcome and death (**Fig. 1**).[10] Use of warfarin increases the risk of hematoma enlargement more than threefold and also increases the duration of risk: the median time to detection of hematoma expansion was 21.4 hours, 2.5 times later in warfarin-treated patients in one study.[11]

Rapid reversal of the anticoagulant effects of warfarin appears to be crucial in preventing hematoma enlargement.[12,13] All major international guidelines for warfarin reversal in ICH include intravenous vitamin K along with some combination of faster-acting agents (prothrombin complex concentrate, fresh frozen plasma, or recombinant factor VIIa).[14] Even when the INR is completely reversed on admission, hematoma enlargement may occur if the INR rises again as the effects of short-acting reversal agents wear off. Retrospective studies and case reports link hematoma enlargement to nonsustained INR correction and suggest that treatment response needs to be sustained for at least 24 hours.[13]

Recurrence Risk of Intracerebral Hemorrhage

In a systematic review of 10 studies encompassing 1880 primary ICH survivors over a mean follow-up of 3.4 years, the ICH recurrence rate was approximately 2.4% per patient-year (95% confidence interval [CI] 2.0%–2.8%).[15] Lobar hemorrhage location

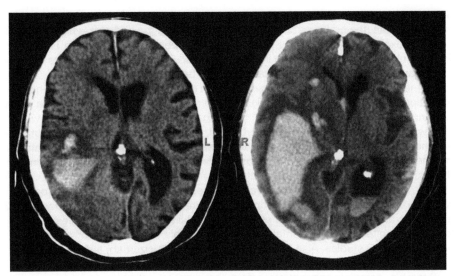

Fig. 1. Head CT scan 1 and 3 hours after the onset of left hemiplegia in a 90-year-old man with hypertension and dementia. The right temporo-occipital ICH demonstrated in the first image has enlarged in the second image, which was obtained because of clinical deterioration. The second image also demonstrates development of intraventricular hemorrhage, new foci of hemorrhage in the right frontal lobe, and worsening midline shift.

was a notable risk factor, conferring a more than twofold higher risk of recurrence relative to deep hemorrhage location (4.4% vs 2.1% per patient-year, $P = .002$). Adding data from a trial restricted to primary lobar ICH, the recurrence rate among survivors of lobar ICH was 5.4% per patient-year (95% CI 4.1%–7.1%). Ischemic stroke during follow-up was less common than ICH at a rate of 1.1% per patient-year (95% CI 0.8%–1.7%).

More recent studies have reported annual ICH recurrence rates of 1.7% to 3.7%, with rates in Western studies (1.7%–2.3%)[16–20] typically lower than those in Asian studies (2.3%–3.7%).[21–23] Factors associated with recurrence included age older than 65 years, lobar ICH location, ICH associated with systemic disease or amyloid angiopathy (cerebral amyloid angiopathy [CAA]), and presence of intraventricular hemorrhage. Ischemic stroke during follow-up was more frequent (1.3%–4.2% per year) than in the earlier systematic review. Recurrence rates are typically highest in the first year, declining thereafter, but in a prospective German cohort study, the risk of any stroke (ischemic or hemorrhagic) after lobar ICH remained higher than 7% over a 3-year period, whereas it decreased from 5.8% at 1 year to 2.9% in subsequent years after deep ICH.[19]

Cerebral microbleeds have been cited as a risk factor for both anticoagulant-associated[24] and antiplatelet-associated[25] ICH. Among warfarin users, the relationship is independent of increased INR and hypertension (odds ratio [OR] 7.38, 95% CI 1.05–51.83). Other clinical and radiographic factors that may predict recurrence of ICH include uncontrolled hypertension[26] and the presence of lacunar infarcts[27] or leukoaraiosis.[28]

Novel Oral Anticoagulants

Although warfarin therapy effectively reduces thromboembolic risk in patients with atrial fibrillation, its drawbacks of increased bleeding risk, drug and food interactions, and requirement of routine monitoring have contributed to undertreatment of at-risk populations and prompted the development of alternative treatments.[29] In the past 5 years, 4 agents (the oral direct thrombin inhibitor dabigatran and oral factor Xa inhibitors rivaroxaban, apixaban, and edoxaban) have been approved by the Food and Drug Administration (FDA) for use in atrial fibrillation. These agents are more convenient than warfarin, have fewer interactions, and have better safety profiles.

In a meta-analysis of 4 trials of these agents in more than 70,000 patients with atrial fibrillation, novel OAC use resulted in a lower risk of intracranial hemorrhage than warfarin use (risk reduction [RR] 0.48).[30] Dabigatran users with ICH fared no worse than warfarin users with ICH in the RE-LY trial,[31] and in a retrospective study of 585 Japanese patients, those with rivaroxaban-associated ICH had smaller hematoma volumes, less hematoma expansion, and lower risk of poor functional outcome or death compared with warfarin-associated ICH.[32]

There are presently no FDA-approved antidotes in the case of bleeding associated with the novel OACs. On the horizon is a recombinant factor Xa derivative, andexanet alfa, which has shown efficacy in reversing bleeding associated with the factor Xa inhibitors in experimental hemorrhage models,[33] and is currently being evaluated in phase 3 studies. Also in phase 3 studies is idarucizumab, a humanized antibody fragment being investigated as an antidote to dabigatran. In the meantime, prothrombin complex concentrate offers the greatest rationale as a nonspecific reversal agent in the case of ICH.[34]

Can Patients Be Anticoagulated After Intracerebral Hemorrhage?

Once the INR is reversed and the patient is out of the high-risk window for hematoma enlargement, the next decision is whether anticoagulation can be resumed. There is considerable controversy regarding this question. In a nationwide Japanese survey of neurospecialists responsible for ICH management, 91% of respondents indicated that they resume anticoagulation after warfarin-associated ICH, 3% switch to antiplatelet therapy, and 6% avoid antithrombotic therapy. Among those who resume anticoagulation, timing was within the first week in 28%, during the second week in 25%, in weeks 3 or 4 in 28%, and after 1 month in 18%.[35] When a group of international experts in clinical stroke, neurologic intensive care, and hematology and coagulation were posed the question of when after ICH to resume anticoagulation in a patient with a prosthetic heart valve, responses ranged from 2 to 14 days.[36] There was no consensus among experts regarding whether warfarin should be restarted for atrial fibrillation, but risk of thromboembolism (based on previous event) and risk of ICH recurrence (based on location of the original hemorrhage) dominated the deliberation.

Clearly the decision of whether or not to anticoagulate hinges on the relative risks of thromboembolism *off* OAC and recurrent ICH *on* OAC. The risk of thromboembolism depends on the underlying condition. We focus on the 2 conditions most frequently observed in the setting of ICH, atrial fibrillation and mechanical heart valves, and also consider venous thromboembolism (VTE) prophylaxis and treatment.

Venous thromboembolism risk in acute intracerebral hemorrhage

Patients with ICH are at increased risk of VTE. Up to 15% of patients with ICH have clinically apparent deep vein thrombosis (DVT); among those with hemiplegia, as many as 40% may have asymptomatic DVT.[37] Fatal pulmonary embolism (PE) occurs in up to 5%, typically after the first week.[38] Intermittent pneumatic compression significantly decreases the incidence of asymptomatic DVT after ICH.[39] Whether the addition of anticoagulation reduces VTE further is not clear; there was no benefit in 2 small randomized trials in which subcutaneous heparin was started on day 4 or 10,[40,41] but in an uncontrolled extension of one study, treatment begun on day 2 reduced VTE incidence.[40]

There are no data on the morbidity and mortality associated with untreated clinical VTE in the setting of ICH, but one estimate puts the risk of fatal clinical PE at 10% to 20% or more and nonfatal clinical PE at 10% to 20% among patients with ICH and untreated DVT, and at 20% to 30% or more and 10% to 20% for those with untreated PE. This is in contrast to risks of 0.3% and 3.9% for treated patients presenting with DVT and 1.7% and 4.1% for treated patients presenting with PE.[42] An additional concern for untreated VTE survivors is development of the post-thrombotic syndrome, which was nearly universal in the pre-anticoagulant era.[43]

There may be a subgroup of patients with nonmassive PE, adequate cardiopulmonary reserve, and negative serial ultrasounds over a 2-week period who have a relatively benign prognosis in the absence of treatment and may be considered for observation only.[44] Otherwise, treatment of VTE is essential. Insertion of an inferior vena cava filter in patients with proximal DVT reduces the likelihood of PE, but is associated with an increased risk of recurrent DVT.[45] In addition, the filter may become thrombosed in 5%,[46] an event that results in PE in one-third.[47]

Thromboembolism risk in patients with atrial fibrillation

Based on summary analysis of 5 primary prevention trials in atrial fibrillation, the annual risk of thromboembolism is 4.5% and is reduced 68% with warfarin.[48] The risk of embolism in a given patient with atrial fibrillation can be refined further using validated clinical prediction rules, such as the $CHADS_2$[49] or CHA_2DS_2-VASc,[50] and may be as high as 18% in those with multiple comorbidities (**Table 1**). No antithrombotic therapy or aspirin is recommended for patients with a low embolic risk ($CHADS_2$ or CHA_2DS_2-VASc 0), whereas oral anticoagulation is recommended for patients at moderate or high risk ($CHADS_2$ or CHA_2DS_2-VASc $\geq$1 or 2). Incorporating contemporary stroke risk estimates and use of novel OACs, anticoagulation may be the preferred treatment above a stroke rate of 0.9% per year.[51]

Thromboembolism risk in patients with mechanical prosthetic heart valves

Based on meta-analysis of 46 studies including more than 13,000 patients, the risk of valve thrombosis associated with a mechanical prosthetic heart valve (MHV) is approximately 1.8 per 100 patient-years and is reduced almost 90% to 0.2 with the use of warfarin. The incidence of major embolism (defined as causing death, residual neurologic deficit, or peripheral ischemia requiring surgery) is approximately 4 per 100 patient-years and is reduced by 80% with warfarin.[52]

Thromboembolic risk associated with an MHV is affected by both patient-related and prosthesis-related factors.[52] Among the patient-related factors are concomitant atrial fibrillation, which increases the embolic risk sevenfold or more, increased chamber size and decreased ventricular function, congestive heart failure, severe mitral stenosis, and a history of previous embolic events.

Prosthesis-related factors include valve position, valve model, and time from surgery. Mitral valve prosthesis is associated with a fivefold greater incidence of valve thrombosis and a 1.5 times greater incidence of embolic events than aortic valve prosthesis, which is likely related to the higher incidence of atrial fibrillation. In a recent population-based cohort study, the incidence of thromboembolism was 1.8 per 100 patient-years in patients with an aortic MHV and 2.2 per 100 patient-years in those with a mitral MHV.[53] This differential embolic risk is reflected in a higher recommended INR target for mitral valve prostheses (2.5–3.5 compared with 2.0–3.0 for aortic).[54] The first-generation prostheses, like the Starr-Edwards cage-ball valve, have the highest thromboembolic risk and therefore a higher recommended INR range of 4.0 to 5.0. Risk associated with tilting disk valves (eg, Bjork-Shiley or Medtronic Hall) and bileaflet

Table 1
Validated clinical prediction rules for estimating the risk of embolism in patients with atrial fibrillation

	CHADS$_2$ Risk Criteria	Points	Total Score	Annual Stroke Risk (%)
C	Congestive heart failure (CHF)	1	0	1.9
H	Hypertension	1	1	2.8
A	Age ≥75 y	1	2	4.0
D	Diabetes mellitus	1	3	5.9
S$_2$	(Prior) Stroke or TIA or thromboembolism	2	4	8.5
			5	12.5
			6	18.2

	CHA$_2$DS$_2$-VASc Risk Criteria	Points	Total Score	Annual Stroke Risk (%)
C	CHF or left ventricular systolic dysfunction	1	0	0
H	Hypertension	1	1	1.3
A$_2$	Age ≥75 y	2	2	2.2
D	Diabetes mellitus	1	3	3.2
S$_2$	(Prior) Stroke or transient ischemic attack	2	4	4.0
V	Vascular disease[a]	1	5	6.7
A	Age 65-74 y	1	6	9.8
Sc	Sex category (i.e., female sex)	1	7	9.6
			8	6.7
			9	15.2

Abbreviation: TIA, transient ischemic attack.
[a] e.g., peripheral artery disease, coronary artery disease, aortic atheroma.
Adapted from Gage BF, Waterman AD, Shannon W, et al. Validation of clinical classification schemes for predicting stroke: results from the National Registry of Atrial Fibrillation. JAMA 2001;285(22):2864–70, with permission; and Lip GY, Nieuwlaat R, Pisters R, et al. Refining clinical risk stratification for predicting stroke and thromboembolism in atrial fibrillation using a novel risk factor-based approach: the Euro Heart Survey on Atrial Fibrillation. Chest 2010;137(2):263–72, with permission.

valves (eg, St Jude Medical) is 30% to 40% lower.[55] Finally, the time interval from valve replacement surgery is important, with the greatest risk being in the first 3 months and 20% of all thromboembolic complications occurring in the first month.

Safety of withholding anticoagulation after intracerebral hemorrhage in patients at high thromboembolic risk
Only one sizable prospective study has evaluated the safety of withholding anticoagulation after ICH in 108 patients at high thromboembolic risk due to atrial fibrillation (56), prosthetic heart valves (30), venous thromboembolism (110), and other causes (11).[56] In this series, 8 thromboembolic events occurred, with a clustering in the first week. The overall rate was 0.66/1000 patient-days at risk. No thromboembolic events occurred among the 25 in whom OAC was resumed after a median of 11 days.

The largest retrospective study involved 141 patients in whom warfarin was discontinued for a median of 10 days after intracranial hemorrhage.[57] Three patients had an ischemic stroke within 30 days of warfarin cessation, all of which occurred during the first week. Kaplan-Meier estimates of the risk of having an ischemic stroke at 30 days after warfarin discontinuation were 2.9% (95% CI 0%–8.0%) for the 52 patients whose indication for anticoagulation was prosthetic heart valve, 2.6% (95% CI 0%–7.6%) for the 53 whose indication was atrial fibrillation/cardioembolic stroke, and 4.8% (95% CI 0%–13.6%) for the 36 whose indication was recurrent cerebrovascular event.

Reviewing data from 63 primarily low-quality studies comprising 492 patients with intracranial hemorrhage while on OAC, Hawryluk and colleagues[58] reported a 6.1% rate of thromboembolic complications after ICH. Of the 30 thromboembolic events, 3 occurred on days 1 to 2, 8 on days 3 to 4, and most of the remainder 10 or more days after ICH. Among the 12 of 30 patients for whom time of anticoagulation restart was specified, two-thirds resumed anticoagulation on day 3 to 10 after ICH. Patients restarting OAC more than 72 hours after ICH were more likely to have a thromboembolic event ($P = .006$).

Retrospective studies in which OACs were withheld chronically in mixed populations (atrial fibrillation, MHV, VTE) report thromboembolism in 20% to 24% of patients over a mean duration of follow-up of 3.5 years.[59,60]

Safety of restarting anticoagulation in the first week after intracerebral hemorrhage
A number of lines of evidence suggest that once hematoma stability has been verified, low-dose anticoagulation can be safely administered. First, continuing anticoagulation in the setting of hemorrhagic conversion of embolic stroke appears to be safe without an increase in hemorrhage or clinical worsening.[61,62] Second, observational[63,64] and randomized controlled trial data[65,66] on the safety of early (0–72 hours after injury) parenteral low-dose anticoagulation for VTE prophylaxis after traumatic brain injury are generally favorable, with no symptomatic hemorrhage progression. A twofold higher rate of hematoma enlargement among patients who received low molecular weight heparin (LMWH) in one study may reflect imbalances in disease severity between the treatment groups.[67]

In the International Stroke Trial, which compared 2 doses of unfractionated heparin equivalent to partial thromboplastin time 30 to 40 or 50 to 60, aspirin, both, or neither within 48 hours of acute stroke, 310 patients were administered heparin whose event was found on postrandomization computed tomography (CT) to have been hemorrhagic (58% primary ICH, 42% hemorrhagic transformation of ischemic stroke). There was a nonsignificant increase in the risk of recurrent ICH during the 2-week treatment period in the heparin group (OR 2.0, 95% CI 0.86–4.70).[68] Of course, because the presence of hemorrhage was not known, there was no verification of hematoma stability before heparin was administered.

Finally, in primary ICH (**Table 2**), 2 small trials demonstrated that starting low-dose heparin after 48 hours does not increase the incidence of hematoma enlargement. In one, 46 patients with ICH were randomized to begin low-dose subcutaneous heparin on the 4th (investigational group) or 10th (control group) day after hemorrhage.[41] When no increase in symptomatic hematoma enlargement was detected, a third nonrandomized group of 22 patients starting heparin on day 2 was added. No instances of symptomatic hematoma enlargement occurred.[40] In the other trial, 75 patients were randomized to subcutaneous enoxaparin or compression stockings 48 hours after ICH. No instances of hematoma enlargement or new hemorrhages were detected on head CT at 72 hours or at 7 or 21 days, including among those who had had hematoma enlargement on their 24-hour scan.[69] Two additional retrospective studies support the safety of low-dose anticoagulation as early as 24 hours after ICH, with no significant increase in the frequency of symptomatic hematoma enlargement.[70,71] In a meta-analysis of these primary ICH trials, there was a nonsignificant reduction in mortality in the treated groups (16.1% vs 20.9%; RR 0.76; 95% CI 0.57–1.03; $P = .07$).[72]

American Heart Association Guidelines recommend that after documentation of cessation of bleeding, low-dose subcutaneous LMWH or unfractionated heparin

Table 2
Clinical studies of low-dose heparin or low molecular weight heparin in the first week after intracerebral hemorrhage

	Dickmann et al,[41] 1988	Boer et al,[40] 1991	Orken et al,[69] 2009	Wasay et al,[70] 2008	Tetri et al,[71] 2008
Study design	Prospective, randomized	Prospective, nonrandomized	Prospective, randomized	Retrospective, nonrandomized	Retrospective, nonrandomized
No. patients	46	68[a]	75	458	407
Treatment	sc UFH	sc UFH	sc LMWH	sc UFH	sc LMWH
Initiation of treatment	4 d	2 d	2 d	1–6 d	1 d
Duration of follow-up	10 d	10 d	21 d	NR	3 mo
Hematoma enlargement diagnosis	Any HE on CT at 1, 6, or 10 d or after clinical worsening	Any HE on CT at 1, 6, or 10 d or after clinical worsening	Any HE on CT at 3, 7, or 21 d	Any HE on CT done for clinical worsening	HE >33% on CT repeated during 1st wk in 284 patients
Hematoma enlargement (treated vs control)	4.3% vs 13.0%	0% vs 8.7%	0% vs 0%	0.5% vs 0%	8.8% vs 7.1%
Death (treated vs control)	21.7% vs 17.4%	9.1% vs 19.6%	NR	12.5% vs 20.2%	19.4% vs 21.1%

Abbreviations: CT, computed tomography; HE, hematoma enlargement; LMWH, low molecular weight heparin; NR, not reported; sc, subcutaneous; UFH, unfractionated heparin.
[a] Includes patients from Dickmann et al,[41] 1988.

may be considered for prevention of VTE in patients with impaired mobility after 1 to 4 days from onset.[73]

Regarding resumption of full-dose anticoagulation, 12 of 144 patients in one study had either intravenous heparin or warfarin started within the first week after ICH. There were no instances of ICH recurrence during hospitalization in these patients (nor in the 23 whose anticoagulation was resumed later in the first month).[57]

In the systematic review of 492 patients with OAC-associated ICH discussed in the last section, 12 recurrent hemorrhages occurred within the first 72 hours, 3 at 3 to 10 days, and none at 10 to 30 days after ICH. Recurrent hemorrhages were more likely to occur in patients whose anticoagulation was started within the first few days.[58]

Safety of long-term anticoagulation after intracerebral hemorrhage

The risk of recurrent ICH in patients who receive vitamin K antagonists after intracranial hemorrhage has been evaluated in 3 prospective studies, with reported spontaneous recurrences in 0% to 9% over 2 years of follow-up. In the largest of these,[74] which included 267 patients with traumatic or spontaneous hemorrhage, anticoagulation was restarted after a median of 60 days. During 778 patient-years of follow-up, intracranial hemorrhage recurred in 20 patients (7.5%; rate 2.56/100 patient-years) at a median of 16.5 months. Considering only the 99 spontaneous intraparenchymal hemorrhages, there were 9 spontaneous recurrences.

In a second study, 48 patients were followed for a mean of 43 months after warfarin-associated ICH. Compared with no recurrences in the 25 patients who did not restart warfarin, 1 recurrent spontaneous ICH and 2 traumatic ICHs occurred in the 23 who restarted warfarin.[60]

The third prospective study reported no recurrences over a mean follow-up of 2 years among 12 patients who received OAC compared with 9 recurrences among 484 who did not receive OAC after ICH.[19]

Last, a systematic review restricted only to patients with a mechanical valve prosthesis and OAC-associated ICH (n = 120) yielded 2 recurrent intracranial hemorrhages after resumption of OAC over a mean follow-up of 7.9 months.[75]

Decision analysis: should anticoagulation be resumed after intracerebral hemorrhage?

Eckman and colleagues[76] used a Markov state transition decision model to try to address whether patients can be anticoagulated after ICH. Based on their model, anticoagulation was predicted to increase both the frequency and severity of future strokes in a hypothetical patient with atrial fibrillation and a lobar hemorrhage. Withholding anticoagulation improved quality-adjusted life expectancy by 1.9 years. They concluded that not anticoagulating is the preferred strategy after lobar ICH unless the rate of recurrent ICH is less than 1.4% per year.

In deep hemispheric ICH, anticoagulation was predicted to yield fewer strokes but with more severe outcome than a strategy of do not anticoagulate. Because of the lower ICH recurrence risk, withholding anticoagulation resulted in a smaller gain of 0.3 quality-adjusted life years. Eckman and colleagues[76] concluded that anticoagulating after deep ICH is preferred only among those at high ischemic stroke risk (>6.5% per year).

These data are limited by the many assumptions used to derive the model. One in particular that may have led to overestimation of the harm of anticoagulation was the assumption of a very high 15% annual rate of recurrence after lobar ICH, which was based on a single study and is much higher than that demonstrated in other studies, including one from the same group.[77]

Novel oral anticoagulants after intracerebral hemorrhage
The role of the novel OACs in the management of patients after OAC-associated ICH has not been studied. Given that the major bleeding risk associated with apixaban in the AVERROES trial was no greater than that of aspirin when administered to patients with atrial fibrillation who were considered not to be warfarin candidates, apixaban might represent an alternative to warfarin after ICH.[78] This strategy remains unproven, however, as serious bleeding with previous warfarin use was the reason for unsuitability of warfarin in only 3% of the patients enrolled in AVERROES. Use of the novel OACs is not indicated as an alternative to warfarin in patients with MHV, given the lack of efficacy and increased bleeding risk associated with dabigatran use in the RE-ALIGN trial.[79]

ANTIPLATELET THERAPY AND INTRACEREBRAL HEMORRHAGE
Background

Meta-analyses of aspirin use for primary and secondary prevention of myocardial infarction and ischemic stroke demonstrate a 15%–34% reduction in mortality, stroke, and myocardial infarction but also a significant increase in the risk of hemorrhagic stroke (12 events per 10,000 persons).[80,81] In the randomized ASA and Carotid Endarterectomy (ACE) trial studying effects of low versus high dose aspirin among patients undergoing carotid endarterectomy,[82] there was a non-significantly higher risk of hemorrhagic stroke in patients in the 650 mg or 1300 mg groups than in the 81 mg or 325 mg groups (RR 1.68; 95% CI, 0.77–3.68, $P = .18$). There was no dose-response relationship between aspirin and risk of hemorrhagic stroke in a meta-analysis, however.[81]

Antiplatelet Therapy and Intracerebral Hemorrhage

There are conflicting data on the effect of previous antiplatelet agent use on hematoma enlargement and clinical outcome after ICH.[83,84] Compared with aspirin use, clopidogrel use may confer greater risk.[85] Platelet dysfunction as measured by platelet function assays has been associated with hematoma expansion and worse outcome,[86] but to date, platelet transfusion has not been demonstrated to provide a mortality benefit or improved functional outcome.[87] Routine use of platelet transfusions in this setting is not recommended by the American Heart Association.[73]

Can Patients Be Restarted on Antiplatelet Therapy After Intracerebral Hemorrhage?

There are no randomized controlled trial data currently available to address the question of safety of resumption of antiplatelet therapy after ICH. The ongoing REstart or STop Antithrombotics Randomised Trial (RESTART, ISRCTN71907627, http://www. RESTARTtrial.org/) is investigating whether a policy of starting antiplatelet therapy after ICH results in a net reduction in serious vascular events compared with a policy of avoiding antiplatelet therapy. Anticipated completion is in 2018. In the meantime, 5 observational studies provide some guidance, although all suffer from probable bias by indication.[19,77,88–90] In 4 of these, aspirin exposure after ICH did not increase the risk of recurrence; only in lobar ICH survivors did one study suggest harm.[77]

Among 56 Chinese patients who resumed aspirin after ICH in a study by Chong and colleagues,[88] there was a twofold reduction in the incidence of combined vascular events (ischemic plus hemorrhagic) compared with 384 who did not resume aspirin (52 per 1000 patient-aspirin years vs 113 per 1000 patient-years, $P = .04$), and there was no difference in the risk of recurrent ICH alone (22.7/1000 patient-aspirin years vs 22.4/1000 patient-aspirin years, $P = .70$).

In a Scottish study, ischemic strokes and myocardial infarctions were more than twice as common as recurrent ICH over a median of 41 months of follow-up among 417 patients with ICH, and antiplatelet exposure in 29% of them did not increase the risk of recurrent ICH (hazard ratio 1.07, 95% CI 0.24–4.84).[89]

In a prospective German study of 496 patients, use of antiplatelet therapy in 28% did not impact risk of ICH recurrence. Of 9 ICH recurrences over a mean follow-up of 2 years, only 1 occurred under use of antiplatelet therapy.[19]

Investigators at Massachusetts General Hospital reported no negative effect of antiplatelet use after ICH in 22% of 207 patients.[90] In a subsequent study by the same group that focused on lobar ICH, aspirin was not associated with ICH recurrence in univariate analysis, but after adjusting for baseline clinical predictors, it independently increased the risk of recurrent ICH (adjusted hazard ratio 3.95, 95% CI 1.6–8.3).[77] However, the cohort of 104 patients included only 16 who had exposure to aspirin during the study period, and the validity of the results have been questioned because of the possibility of overfitting of the multivariable model.[91]

In the International Stroke Trial described previously and the Chinese Acute Stroke Trial, in which patients were randomized to aspirin 160 mg or placebo within 48 hours of stroke onset, 398 patients allocated to aspirin were subsequently found to have had ICH on postrandomization CT. There was no increase in the risk of recurrent ICH during the 2-week treatment period in the aspirin group (OR 1.02, 95% CI 0.58–1.79).[68]

Decisions about whether to resume antiplatelet therapy after ICH require an assessment of the risk-benefit ratio, just as should occur for individuals being considered for antiplatelet therapy in primary or secondary cardiovascular and cerebrovascular disease prevention in the absence of a previous hemorrhagic event. Known factors that increase the risk for ICH during antiplatelet use include previous stroke and a history of hypertension, which are notably the same factors that confer the greatest need for antiplatelet therapy. Other risk factors for bleeding may include age, race, bleeding disorders, leukoaraiosis, and underlying lesion (eg, neoplasm, aneurysm, vascular malformation, arteritis, CAA).[92]

Decision analysis
Based on the same Markov decision model described earlier,[76] aspirin was found to be the preferred treatment among patients with deep ICH who had intermediate ischemic stroke risk and recurrent ICH relative risk less than approximately 1.3. Among patients with lobar ICH, aspirin was preferred when the risk of ischemic stroke was average (4.5% per year) and the relative risk of recurrent ICH was less than approximately 1.04.

SUMMARY

Decisions about whether to resume antithrombotic therapy after ICH require individual assessment of the risk of thromboembolism versus risk of recurrent ICH (**Table 3**). No randomized controlled trials provide direction; no studies provide an accurate assessment of the risk of ICH recurrence when antithrombotic therapy is restarted; and in most cases, guidelines and consensus statements are not available. First and foremost, estimation of the risk of thromboembolism off antithrombotic therapy should consider the indication for therapy, with treatment typically most justified in the setting of secondary prevention versus primary prevention and in the management of patients with mechanical heart valve prosthesis or symptomatic venous thromboembolism (Category T4). Patients with atrial fibrillation can be risk stratified with the use of simple tools, such as the $CHADS_2$ or CHA_2DS_2-VASc. Estimation of the risk of recurrent ICH should consider ICH location, patient age and ethnicity, underlying systemic disease, presence of microbleeds, and probability of CAA. The higher risk associated with lobar

Table 3
Risk-benefit analysis for resuming antithrombotic therapy after intracerebral hemorrhage (ICH)

Factors Increasing Risk of Thromboembolism		Factors Increasing Risk of ICH Recurrence
Highest Risk	Moderately High Risk	
Mechanical valve prosthesis • Mitral position • First-generation model • With concomitant atrial fibrillation, congestive heart failure, severe mitral stenosis, or previous embolic event • Placement within previous 3 mo Atrial fibrillation with previous stroke Proximal deep venous thrombosis or pulmonary embolism	Aortic mechanical valve prosthesis Atrial fibrillation without previous stroke but with $CHADS_2$ or CHA_2DS_2-VASc $\geq$1 or 2 Multiple previous ischemic events (cerebral, coronary, or systemic)	Lobar ICH location Cerebral amyloid angiopathy Age >65 y Asian ethnicity Uncontrolled hypertension Bleeding diathesis (eg, liver failure, hemophilia) Cerebral microbleeds seen on gradient-echo MRI

ICH location, age older than 65 years, uncontrolled hypertension, bleeding diathesis, previous microbleeds, and probable CAA may outweigh the benefit of treatment in these situations (Category T4). Although use of the novel OACs may offer an appealing alternative in the setting of atrial fibrillation or VTE given their lower ICH risk compared with warfarin, this strategy remains unproven. The impact of antiplatelet therapy on ICH risk is generally less than that of anticoagulant therapy, so in some cases, antiplatelet therapy offers a reasonable compromise (Category T4).

When OAC resumption is judged to be indicated, the timing of when to restart is controversial, and little guidance is provided by high-quality prospective studies. Low-dose subcutaneous unfractionated and LMWHs are likely safe for use in VTE prophylaxis in ICH after the first 24 to 48 hours when cessation of bleeding has been documented (Category T2). Low-quality data suggest the optimal start time for full-dose anticoagulation may be 3 to 5 days after ICH; expert opinion is divided, often with a favoring of 7 to 14 days or more after ICH. Decisions should be individualized based on any high-risk features favoring thromboembolism or rehemorrhage, but a reasonable approach may be to resume full-dose OAC by 7 days because the available data suggest a moderately low risk of thromboembolic complications during this time period for the highest risk patients with prosthetic valves (Category T4). In any patients restarted on warfarin, additional pragmatic strategies to lower the risk of recurrent ICH include targeting the lowest efficacious INR, vigilant INR monitoring to avoid excessive anticoagulation, and aggressive blood pressure control.

REFERENCES

1. Franke CL, van Swieten JC, Algra A, et al. Prognostic factors in patients with intracerebral haematoma. J Neurol Neurosurg Psychiatry 1992;55(8):653–7.
2. Fang MC, Go AS, Chang Y, et al. Death and disability from warfarin-associated intracranial and extracranial hemorrhages. Am J Med 2007;120(8):700–5.
3. Shen AY, Yao JF, Brar SS, et al. Racial/ethnic differences in the risk of intracranial hemorrhage among patients with atrial fibrillation. J Am Coll Cardiol 2007;50(4): 309–15.

4. Hankey GJ, Stevens SR, Piccini JP, et al. Intracranial hemorrhage among patients with atrial fibrillation anticoagulated with warfarin or rivaroxaban: the rivaroxaban once daily, oral, direct factor Xa inhibition compared with vitamin K antagonism for prevention of stroke and embolism trial in atrial fibrillation. Stroke 2014; 45(5):1304–12.
5. Shireman TI, Howard PA, Kresowik TF, et al. Combined anticoagulant-antiplatelet use and major bleeding events in elderly atrial fibrillation patients. Stroke 2004; 35(10):2362–7.
6. Hart RG, Benavente O, Pearce LA. Increased risk of intracranial hemorrhage when aspirin is combined with warfarin: a meta-analysis and hypothesis. Cerebrovasc Dis 1999;9(4):215–7.
7. Fang MC, Chang Y, Hylek EM, et al. Advanced age, anticoagulation intensity, and risk for intracranial hemorrhage among patients taking warfarin for atrial fibrillation. Ann Intern Med 2004;141(10):745–52.
8. Berwaerts J, Dijkhuizen RS, Robb OJ, et al. Prediction of functional outcome and in-hospital mortality after admission with oral anticoagulant-related intracerebral hemorrhage. Stroke 2000;31(11):2558–62.
9. Hart RG. What causes intracerebral hemorrhage during warfarin therapy? Neurology 2000;55(7):907–8.
10. Brott T, Broderick J, Kothari R, et al. Early hemorrhage growth in patients with intracerebral hemorrhage. Stroke 1997;28(1):1–5.
11. Flibotte JJ, Hagan N, O'Donnell J, et al. Warfarin, hematoma expansion, and outcome of intracerebral hemorrhage. Neurology 2004;63(6):1059–64.
12. Huttner HB, Schellinger PD, Hartmann M, et al. Hematoma growth and outcome in treated neurocritical care patients with intracerebral hemorrhage related to oral anticoagulant therapy: comparison of acute treatment strategies using vitamin K, fresh frozen plasma, and prothrombin complex concentrates. Stroke 2006;37(6): 1465–70.
13. Yasaka M, Minematsu K, Naritomi H, et al. Predisposing factors for enlargement of intracerebral hemorrhage in patients treated with warfarin. Thromb Haemost 2003;89(2):278–83.
14. Goldstein JN, Rosand J, Schwamm LH. Warfarin reversal in anticoagulant-associated intracerebral hemorrhage. Neurocrit Care 2008;9(2):277–83.
15. Bailey RD, Hart RG, Benavente O, et al. Recurrent brain hemorrhage is more frequent than ischemic stroke after intracranial hemorrhage. Neurology 2001;56:773–7.
16. Vermeer SE, Algra A, Franke CL, et al. Long-term prognosis after recovery from primary intracerebral hemorrhage. Neurology 2002;59(2):205–9.
17. Hanger HC, Wilkinson TJ, Fayez-Iskander N, et al. The risk of recurrent stroke after intracerebral haemorrhage. J Neurol Neurosurg Psychiatry 2007;78(8):836–40.
18. Zia E, Engstrom G, Svensson PJ, et al. Three-year survival and stroke recurrence rates in patients with primary intracerebral hemorrhage. Stroke 2009;40(11): 3567–73.
19. Weimar C, Benemann J, Terborg C, et al. Recurrent stroke after lobar and deep intracerebral hemorrhage: a hospital-based cohort study. Cerebrovasc Dis 2011; 32(3):283–8.
20. Huhtakangas J, Lopponen P, Tetri S, et al. Predictors for recurrent primary intracerebral hemorrhage: a retrospective population-based study. Stroke 2013;44(3): 585–90.
21. Inagawa T, Ohbayashi N, Takechi A, et al. Primary intracerebral hemorrhage in Izumo City, Japan: incidence rates and outcome in relation to the site of hemorrhage. Neurosurgery 2003;53(6):1283–97.

22. Yokota C, Minematsu K, Hasegawa Y, et al. Long-term prognosis, by stroke subtypes, after a first-ever stroke: a hospital-based study over a 20-year period. Cerebrovasc Dis 2004;18(2):111–6.
23. Yeh SJ, Tang SC, Tsai LK, et al. Pathogenetical subtypes of recurrent intracerebral hemorrhage: designations by SMASH-U classification system. Stroke 2014;45(9):2636–42.
24. Ueno H, Naka H, Ohshita T, et al. Association between cerebral microbleeds on T2*-weighted MR images and recurrent hemorrhagic stroke in patients treated with warfarin following ischemic stroke. AJNR Am J Neuroradiol 2008;29(8):1483–6.
25. Naka H, Nomura E, Kitamura J, et al. Antiplatelet therapy as a risk factor for microbleeds in intracerebral hemorrhage patients: analysis using specific antiplatelet agents. J Stroke Cerebrovasc Dis 2013;22(6):834–40.
26. Chen ST, Chiang CY, Hsu CY, et al. Recurrent hypertensive intracerebral hemorrhage. Acta Neurol Scand 1995;91(2):128–32.
27. de JG, Kessels F, Lodder J. Two types of lacunar infarcts: further arguments from a study on prognosis. Stroke 2002;33(8):2072–6.
28. Smith EE, Gurol ME, Eng JA, et al. White matter lesions, cognition, and recurrent hemorrhage in lobar intracerebral hemorrhage. Neurology 2004;63(9):1606–12.
29. Zimetbaum PJ, Thosani A, Yu HT, et al. Are atrial fibrillation patients receiving warfarin in accordance with stroke risk? Am J Med 2010;123(5):446–53.
30. Ruff CT, Giugliano RP, Braunwald E, et al. Comparison of the efficacy and safety of new oral anticoagulants with warfarin in patients with atrial fibrillation: a meta-analysis of randomised trials. Lancet 2014;383(9921):955–62.
31. Connolly SJ, Ezekowitz MD, Yusuf S, et al. Dabigatran versus warfarin in patients with atrial fibrillation. N Engl J Med 2009;361(12):1139–51.
32. Hagii J, Tomita H, Metoki N, et al. Characteristics of intracerebral hemorrhage during rivaroxaban treatment: comparison with those during warfarin. Stroke 2014;45(9):2805–7.
33. Lu G, DeGuzman FR, Hollenbach SJ, et al. A specific antidote for reversal of anticoagulation by direct and indirect inhibitors of coagulation factor Xa. Nat Med 2013;19(4):446–51.
34. Fukuda T, Honda Y, Kamisato C, et al. Reversal of anticoagulant effects of edoxaban, an oral, direct factor Xa inhibitor, with haemostatic agents. Thromb Haemost 2012;107(2):253–9.
35. Maeda K, Koga M, Okada Y, et al. Nationwide survey of neuro-specialists' opinions on anticoagulant therapy after intracerebral hemorrhage in patients with atrial fibrillation. J Neurol Sci 2012;312(1-2):82–5.
36. Aguilar MI, Hart RG, Kase CS, et al. Treatment of warfarin-associated intracerebral hemorrhage: literature review and expert opinion. Mayo Clin Proc 2007;82(1):82–92.
37. Ogata T, Yasaka M, Wakugawa Y, et al. Deep venous thrombosis after acute intracerebral hemorrhage. J Neurol Sci 2008;272(1–2):83–6.
38. Counsell C, Boonyakarnkul S, Dennis M, et al. Primary intracerebral haemorrhage in the Oxfordshire Community Stroke Project; 2. Prognosis. Cerebrovasc Dis 1995;5:26–34.
39. Lacut K, Bressollette L, Le Gal G, et al. Prevention of venous thrombosis in patients with acute intracerebral hemorrhage. Neurology 2005;65(6):865–9.
40. Boeer A, Voth E, Henze T, et al. Early heparin therapy in patients with spontaneous intracerebral haemorrhage. J Neurol Neurosurg Psychiatry 1991;54(5):466–7.
41. Dickmann U, Voth E, Schicha H, et al. Heparin therapy, deep-vein thrombosis and pulmonary embolism after intracerebral hemorrhage. Klin Wochenschr 1988;66(23):1182–3.

42. Kelly J, Hunt BJ, Lewis RR, et al. Anticoagulation or inferior vena cava filter placement for patients with primary intracerebral hemorrhage developing venous thromboembolism? Stroke 2003;34(12):2999–3005.
43. Zilliacus H. On the specific treatment of thrombosis and pulmonary embolism with anticoagulants, with a particular reference to the post thrombotic sequelae. Acta Med Scand 1946;171:1–221.
44. Hull RD, Raskob GE, Ginsberg JS, et al. A noninvasive strategy for the treatment of patients with suspected pulmonary embolism. Arch Intern Med 1994;154(3): 289–97.
45. Decousus H, Leizorovicz A, Parent F, et al. A clinical trial of vena caval filters in the prevention of pulmonary embolism in patients with proximal deep-vein thrombosis. Prevention du Risque d'Embolie Pulmonaire par Interruption Cave Study Group. N Engl J Med 1998;338(7):409–15.
46. Becker DM, Philbrick JT, Selby JB. Inferior vena cava filters. Indications, safety, effectiveness. Arch Intern Med 1992;152(10):1985–94.
47. Tardy B, Mismetti P, Page Y, et al. Symptomatic inferior vena cava filter thrombosis: clinical study of 30 consecutive cases. Eur Respir J 1996;9(10):2012–6.
48. Risk factors for stroke and efficacy of antithrombotic therapy in atrial fibrillation. Analysis of pooled data from five randomized controlled trials. Arch Intern Med 1994;154(13):1449–57.
49. Gage BF, Waterman AD, Shannon W, et al. Validation of clinical classification schemes for predicting stroke: results from the National Registry of Atrial Fibrillation. JAMA 2001;285(22):2864–70.
50. Lip GY, Nieuwlaat R, Pisters R, et al. Refining clinical risk stratification for predicting stroke and thromboembolism in atrial fibrillation using a novel risk factor-based approach: the Euro Heart Survey on Atrial Fibrillation. Chest 2010; 137(2):263–72.
51. Eckman MH, Singer DE, Rosand J, et al. Moving the tipping point: the decision to anticoagulate patients with atrial fibrillation. Circ Cardiovasc Qual Outcomes 2011;4(1):14–21.
52. Cannegieter SC, Rosendaal FR, Briet E. Thromboembolic and bleeding complications in patients with mechanical heart valve prostheses. Circulation 1994; 89(2):635–41.
53. Labaf A, Grzymala-Lubanski B, Stagmo M, et al. Thromboembolism, major bleeding and mortality in patients with mechanical heart valves—a population-based cohort study. Thromb Res 2014;134(2):354–9.
54. Whitlock RP, Sun JC, Fremes SE, et al. Antithrombotic and thrombolytic therapy for valvular disease: antithrombotic therapy and prevention of thrombosis, 9th ed: American College of Chest Physicians evidence-based clinical practice guidelines. Chest 2012;141(2 Suppl):e576S–600S.
55. Cannegieter SC, Rosendaal FR, Wintzen AR, et al. Optimal oral anticoagulant therapy in patients with mechanical heart valves. N Engl J Med 1995;333(1):11–7.
56. De VS, Van CF, van LJ, et al. Risk analysis of thrombo-embolic and recurrent bleeding events in the management of intracranial haemorrhage due to oral anticoagulation. Acta Chir Belg 2005;105(3):268–74.
57. Phan TG, Koh M, Wijdicks EF. Safety of discontinuation of anticoagulation in patients with intracranial hemorrhage at high thromboembolic risk. Arch Neurol 2000;57(12):1710–3.
58. Hawryluk GW, Austin JW, Furlan JC, et al. Management of anticoagulation following central nervous system hemorrhage in patients with high thromboembolic risk. J Thromb Haemost 2010;8(7):1500–8.

59. Gathier CS, Algra A, Rinkel GJ, et al. Long-term outcome after anticoagulation-associated intracerebral haemorrhage with or without restarting antithrombotic therapy. Cerebrovasc Dis 2013;36(1):33–7.
60. Claassen DO, Kazemi N, Zubkov AY, et al. Restarting anticoagulation therapy after warfarin-associated intracerebral hemorrhage. Arch Neurol 2008;65(10): 1313–8.
61. Chamorro A, Vila N, Saiz A, et al. Early anticoagulation after large cerebral embolic infarction: a safety study. Neurology 1995;45(5):861–5.
62. Kim JT, Heo SH, Park MS, et al. Use of antithrombotics after hemorrhagic transformation in acute ischemic stroke. PLoS One 2014;9(2):e89798.
63. Koehler DM, Shipman J, Davidson MA, et al. Is early venous thromboembolism prophylaxis safe in trauma patients with intracranial hemorrhage. J Trauma 2011;70(2):324–9.
64. Farooqui A, Hiser B, Barnes SL, et al. Safety and efficacy of early thromboembolism chemoprophylaxis after intracranial hemorrhage from traumatic brain injury. J Neurosurg 2013;119(6):1576–82.
65. Phelan HA, Wolf SE, Norwood SH, et al. A randomized, double-blinded, placebo-controlled pilot trial of anticoagulation in low-risk traumatic brain injury: the Delayed Versus Early Enoxaparin Prophylaxis I (DEEP I) study. J Trauma Acute Care Surg 2012;73(6):1434–41.
66. Kurtoglu M, Yanar H, Bilsel Y, et al. Venous thromboembolism prophylaxis after head and spinal trauma: intermittent pneumatic compression devices versus low molecular weight heparin. World J Surg 2004;28(8):807–11.
67. Kwiatt ME, Patel MS, Ross SE, et al. Is low-molecular-weight heparin safe for venous thromboembolism prophylaxis in patients with traumatic brain injury? A Western Trauma Association multicenter study. J Trauma Acute Care Surg 2012;73(3):625–8.
68. Keir SL, Wardlaw JM, Sandercock PA, et al. Antithrombotic therapy in patients with any form of intracranial haemorrhage: a systematic review of the available controlled studies. Cerebrovasc Dis 2002;14(3–4):197–206.
69. Orken DN, Kenangil G, Ozkurt H, et al. Prevention of deep venous thrombosis and pulmonary embolism in patients with acute intracerebral hemorrhage. Neurologist 2009;15(6):329–31.
70. Wasay M, Khan S, Zaki KS, et al. A non-randomized study of safety and efficacy of heparin for DVT prophylaxis in intracerebral haemorrhage. J Pak Med Assoc 2008;58(7):362–4.
71. Tetri S, Hakala J, Juvela S, et al. Safety of low-dose subcutaneous enoxaparin for the prevention of venous thromboembolism after primary intracerebral haemorrhage. Thromb Res 2008;123(2):206–12.
72. Paciaroni M, Agnelli G, Venti M, et al. Efficacy and safety of anticoagulants in the prevention of venous thromboembolism in patients with acute cerebral hemorrhage: a meta-analysis of controlled studies. J Thromb Haemost 2011;9(5):893–8.
73. Morgenstern LB, Hemphill JC III, Anderson C, et al. Guidelines for the management of spontaneous intracerebral hemorrhage: a guideline for healthcare professionals from the American Heart Association/American Stroke Association. Stroke 2010;41(9):2108–29.
74. Poli D, Antonucci E, Dentali F, et al. Recurrence of ICH after resumption of anticoagulation with VK antagonists: CHIRONE study. Neurology 2014;82(12):1020–6.
75. Romualdi E, Micieli E, Ageno W, et al. Oral anticoagulant therapy in patients with mechanical heart valve and intracranial haemorrhage. A systematic review. Thromb Haemost 2009;101(2):290–7.

76. Eckman MH, Rosand J, Knudsen KA, et al. Can patients be anticoagulated after intracerebral hemorrhage? A decision analysis. Stroke 2003;34(7):1710–6.
77. Biffi A, Halpin A, Towfighi A, et al. Aspirin and recurrent intracerebral hemorrhage in cerebral amyloid angiopathy. Neurology 2010;75(8):693–8.
78. Connolly SJ, Eikelboom J, Joyner C, et al. Apixaban in patients with atrial fibrillation. N Engl J Med 2011;364(9):806–17.
79. Eikelboom JW, Connolly SJ, Brueckmann M, et al. Dabigatran versus warfarin in patients with mechanical heart valves. N Engl J Med 2013;369(13):1206–14.
80. Collaborative overview of randomised trials of antiplatelet therapy—I: prevention of death, myocardial infarction, and stroke by prolonged antiplatelet therapy in various categories of patients. Antiplatelet Trialists' Collaboration. BMJ 1994; 308(6921):81–106.
81. He J, Whelton PK, Vu B, et al. Aspirin and risk of hemorrhagic stroke: a meta-analysis of randomized controlled trials. JAMA 1998;280(22):1930–5.
82. Taylor DW, Barnett HJ, Haynes RB, et al. Low-dose and high-dose acetylsalicylic acid for patients undergoing carotid endarterectomy: a randomised controlled trial. ASA and Carotid Endarterectomy (ACE) Trial Collaborators. Lancet 1999; 353(9171):2179–84.
83. Sansing LH, Messe SR, Cucchiara BL, et al. Prior antiplatelet use does not affect hemorrhage growth or outcome after ICH. Neurology 2009;72(16):1397–402.
84. Toyoda K, Okada Y, Minematsu K, et al. Antiplatelet therapy contributes to acute deterioration of intracerebral hemorrhage. Neurology 2005;65(7):1000–4.
85. Campbell PG, Yadla S, Sen AN, et al. Emergency reversal of clopidogrel in the setting of spontaneous intracerebral hemorrhage. World Neurosurg 2011; 76(1-2):100–4.
86. Naidech AM, Jovanovic B, Liebling S, et al. Reduced platelet activity is associated with early clot growth and worse 3-month outcome after intracerebral hemorrhage. Stroke 2009;40(7):2398–401.
87. Martin M, Conlon LW. Does platelet transfusion improve outcomes in patients with spontaneous or traumatic intracerebral hemorrhage? Ann Emerg Med 2013; 61(1):58–61.
88. Chong BH, Chan KH, Pong V, et al. Use of aspirin in Chinese after recovery from primary intracranial haemorrhage. Thromb Haemost 2012;107(2):241–7.
89. Flynn RW, MacDonald TM, Murray GD, et al. Prescribing antiplatelet medicine and subsequent events after intracerebral hemorrhage. Stroke 2010;41(11): 2606–11.
90. Viswanathan A, Rakich SM, Engel C, et al. Antiplatelet use after intracerebral hemorrhage. Neurology 2006;66(2):206–9.
91. Al-Shahi SR, Dennis MS. Antiplatelet therapy may be continued after intracerebral hemorrhage. Stroke 2014;45(10):3149–50.
92. Gorelick PB, Weisman SM. Risk of hemorrhagic stroke with aspirin use: an update. Stroke 2005;36(8):1801–7.

Management of Unbled Brain Arteriovenous Malformation Study

J.P. Mohr, MD, MS*, Shadi Yaghi, MD

KEYWORDS

- Arteriovenous malformation • Nonhemorrhagic presentation
- Randomized clinical trial • Interventional management • Medical management

KEY POINTS

- The Unruptured Brain Arteriovenous malformations (ARUBA) is the only randomized clinical trial comparing medical only versus medical plus intervention limited to those patients deemed by participating centers suitable for attempted eradication.
- The death/stroke outcomes led to a recommendation from a National Institute of Neurological Disorders and Stroke (NINDS)-appointed Data and Safety Monitoring Board to halt randomization owing to superiority for the medical arm.
- The NINDS Study Section and Council decided against funding for further follow-up, citing the likelihood the disparities between the medical and interventional arms would persist for the planned additional 5 years of follow-up.

INTRODUCTION

Incidence

In the Cooperative Study of Subarachnoid Hemorrhage, still the largest such series to date, symptomatic arteriovenous malformation (AVMs) were found in 549 of 6368 cases, representing an incidence of 8.6% of subarachnoid hemorrhages.[1] Because subarachnoid hemorrhage accounts for roughly 10% of strokes, AVMs make up approximately 1% of all stroke, or 1.8% in an eligible population of 100,000 studied over a period of 3 years%.[2]

Prevalence

Data on the prevalence of AVMs is difficult to obtain. Early autopsy studies suggested a prevalence of 4.3%.[3] Noninvasive brain imaging has created an increased

Disclosures: ARUBA trial NINDS (NIH) U01 NS051483 (J.P. Mohr); None (S. Yaghi).
Department of Neurology, Doris & Stanley Tananbaum Stroke Center, Neurological Institute, Columbia University Medical Center, 710 West 168th Street, New York, NY 10032, USA
* Corresponding author.
E-mail address: jpm10@columbia.edu

Neurol Clin 33 (2015) 347–359
http://dx.doi.org/10.1016/j.ncl.2014.12.006
0733-8619/15/$ – see front matter © 2015 Elsevier Inc. All rights reserved.

awareness of AVMs over the past few decades. The New York Island Study of a population approximating the 10 million living in Manhattan, Staten Island, Brooklyn, Queens, and Nassau and Suffolk Counties documented 1.34 per 100,000 person-years (95% CI, 1.18–1.49). Hemorrhage is the presenting feature in 0.68 per 100,000 (95% CI, 0.57–0.79).[4] Similar data were published from the population-based Scottish Vascular Malformation Study.[5]

Vascular Features

AVMs are a coiled mass of arteries and veins partially separated by thin islands of sclerotic tissue, lying in a bed formed by displacement rather than invasion of normal brain tissue.[3] Long considered congenital, recent reports document de novo cases.[6] It remains unknown which ones continue to develop and which are status anomalies. No method has been generally agreed on for defining the epicenter of an AVM.[7] There is no special predilection for AVMs in any part of the brain, the locations reflecting the relative volume of the brain represented by a given region.[6] Location seems to have no bearing on the tendency for hemorrhage, growth, regression, vascular complexity, or size. The vast majority of AVMs are single, but noninvasive imaging has increased the number of multiple AVMs, with 1 series citing 9%.[8] When multiple, the lesions are usually small. Growth, stability, and even regression have been documented.[9–11]

Natural History

Before modern imaging, so few cases were discovered incidental to formal angiogram that no useful prognostic data existed. Early estimates of the annual morbidity and mortality of brain AVMs (bAVMs) came from large referral institutions.[12–14] Review of these classic works, whose case material is based mainly on angiographic studies, suggest that their estimates of hemorrhage incidence, morbidity, and mortality were drawn largely from those who came to clinical attention from the subset of the population at greatest risk for hemorrhage, and they did not discover the larger subpopulation of those unaffected or suffering only minor syndromes from hemorrhage.

Ignorance of the natural history of bAVMs has long confounded pretrial, center-based registry data. The widely cited 1990 publication entitled "The natural history of symptomatic arteriovenous malformations of the brain: a 24-year follow-up assessment" was a case series of bAVMs discovered from 1942 to 1975. It cited annual hemorrhage rates as high as 4% and mortality of 1%.[14] The authors pointed out that the majority of the patients (160 of 242) had bled. A surviving co-author commented privately that these cases were considered too daunting for attempted surgical removal. These data may well apply to their cohort, but provide little insight into the true natural history for those discovered with no prior hemorrhage and who are to be followed for annual status with no plan for intervention unless hemorrhage occurs. Even the most recent meta-analyses have been confounded by the inability to segregate those bled from those not, leaving unclear whether the wide range of adverse outcomes from attempts at eradication applies equally to the 2 groups.[15] Few reports have made reference to the treatment outcome segregating with or without pretreatment hemorrhage.[16–18] The difficulties in demonstrating the value of intervention in unbled bAVMs prompted the suggestion such therapy was experimental, despite its being well established.[19]

These percentages have long been used as a basis for treatment to prevent recurrent hemorrhage, and even to prevent initial hemorrhage. Although the most commonly cited "natural history" publication reported relatively high hemorrhage rates, some reports from small populations have documented rates that are even higher.[20,21] Acting on such presumed natural history, young individuals were (and some still are) told that they have a 40% to 50% risk of some major incapacitating or fatal hemorrhage from an AVM in their projected life span. This projection is often made regardless of whether the patient presents with seizure, migraine, unrelated symptoms, or owing to discovery of the bAVM for brain imaging done in pursuit of another diagnosis.

Modern assessments, using noninvasive imaging, have reported much lower rates for those discovered not having bled, some as low as 1% per year.[22–24] Data drawn from a population of almost 9 million persons living in Manhattan, Staten, and Long Island in 2001 through 2004[4] have also modified downward estimates for both initial morbidity and mortality.[4,24–26] Similar findings were reported from the Scottish Vascular Malformation Study[5] and replicated in recent meta-analyses.[27] These studies challenged the basis for intervention in unruptured bAVMs. They were the basis for application for a randomized, clinical trial comparing outcome for those discovered unbled and treated only medically versus those treated medically and also by intervention to eradicate the bAVM.

CLINICAL PRESENTATIONS
Hemorrhage

Hemorrhage is the presenting compliant in approximately one-half of the cases.[28] Primarily parenchymatous hemorrhage occurs most often (63% of cases). Primarily parenchymatous and associated subarachnoid hemorrhage occurs in 32%, and ventricular hemorrhage alone least often, at 6%.[1] For the hemorrhages limited to the parenchyma, the syndrome is a combination of the hemorrhage into the region of the bAVMs with secondary effect on adjacent parenchyma.[29] This secondary effect is often minor, with satisfactory remission of the syndrome.[30] The hemorrhage affecting the subarachnoid space usually involves the convexity, far less often the region of the base of the brain. Vasospasm is uncommon.[31] Because many bAVMs drain to the ventricular wall, the effect of the hemorrhage may primarily be its venting into the ventricular space. A distinctive clinical feature of such ventricular hemorrhages is an unrelenting course over minutes from the onset of headache to stupor. The ventricular hemorrhage usually produces a hemohydrocephalus with limited parenchymal component. If severe, a ventricular drain can be used, but many are mild enough that such drainage can be avoided.

Headache

Headache is a presenting feature in 15% of bAVMs. In 1940, Northfield[32] suggested that recurrent unilateral headache could mean an underlying bAVM. No evidence was presented, but the idea continues to the present day. Headache is such a common complaint in the population at large that it has proved difficult to determine whether the headache associated with AVMs is distinctive in any of its clinical features, including location.[2,27,32] Mackenzie[33] emphasized the tendency of the headaches to occur before the aura and for the aura to persist beyond the few minutes that typifies migraine, a finding not confirmed by others. The literature remains limited; Lees[34] had only 3 cases whose headache was ipsilateral to the AVM among the 11 headache cases in his series of 70 AVMs. More recent authors claim a correlation between headache and AVMs,[35] including occipital location,[36] but others not.[6]

Seizures

Seizures as the presenting complaint affect roughly one-third of bAVMs. The prevalence is greatest in those with bAVMs affecting the convexity.[37] Reports vary widely for severity, ease of control with medication, and prognosis for hemorrhage. Seizures are most common in bAVMs involving the surface of the brain, especially the centro-parietal area,[28] but is unusual for deep AVMs. The type of seizure is often unreported but, where described, focal spells predominate, varying from 45% to 59%.[14] Hemorrhage from bAVM has been found to confer a greater risk for first-ever seizures compared with incidental bAVMs.[38] Seizures are not a prognostic factor for hemorrhage. Hemorrhage occurred within 1 year in only 15% of 90 cases of seizure in the Cooperative Study and their incidence or recurrence is not modified by intervention to eradicate the bAVM.[39]

Cerebral Steal

Roughly 6% of patients with AVM have some focal neurologic deficits of gradual onset. In most, the deficit is limited to the region of the brain served by the AVM. Early angiography showing the dense concentration of contrast flowing through the fistula and the comparatively thinner appearance of nonaffected local vessels supported the idea there could be cerebral steal with ischemia.[40] The reported neurologic syndromes have evolved over periods as short as 3 or as long as 10 years, but with no sudden loss of function to suggest infarction and without obvious instances of hemorrhage. The inferred presence of steal was used to justify intervention to eradicate the bAVM. A publication challenging the role of cerebral steal was based on 32 cases with measurements of feeding arterial pressure showing no ischemic effects in perilesional vessel, and a clinical series of 152, with 13 focal neurologic deficits unrelated to hemorrhage.[41] After publication, a single criticism was published,[42] and cerebral steal reports in case series fell into the low single digits. However, neuropsychological impairments exist and can show improvement in the setting of dural fistulas.[43] Mass effects, mostly in brainstem bAVMs, apply in most cases.[44]

INTERVENTIONAL MANAGEMENT

Center-based registry reports focused on outcomes from intervention have regularly provided demographics of those treated (eg, age, gender, lesion size and location, and usually the percent of the cohort having had prior hemorrhage), but detailed the results of treatment without segregating the outcomes based on pretreatment hemorrhage status.[15] Investigators found it impossible to assess the extent to which the intervention created a clinical disturbance not present before, aggravated one already present, or had no such effects.[45] This publication tendency persists to the present day, despite the awareness that the trial was comparing the outcomes for those bled or not bled. An overview of outcomes was reported in the largest meta-analysis to date (**Fig. 1**).[15]

Treatments to eradicate a bAVM began with surgery. At first, there were attempts to ligate feeding arteries and, in recent years, attempts at complete removal of the lesion. Brain AVMs are embedded in the brain and often associated with deep draining veins, making surgical removal among the most challenging of the neurosurgical procedures. Commonly cited risk factors for surgical eradication are less than 2% for mortality and 5% for significant morbidity, with 12% for minor morbidity after total obliteration of the lesion. Such rates apply mainly to those of small size (<3 cm), no deep venous drainage, and location away from functionally important brain areas, grade I of VI on the Spetzler–Martin grading system.[46] Those of a higher grade can be expected to show higher rates of adverse outcomes. A recent addition has been made to this grading system.[47]

In recent decades, embolization has become popular. It was begun both in hopes of reducing the size of the bAVM to one suitable for surgery, and concerns for

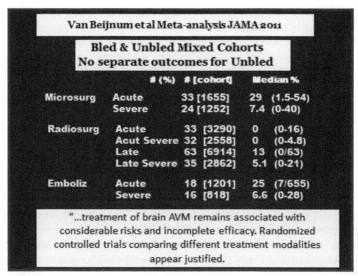

Fig. 1. Meta-analysis reported by Van Beijnum and colleagues in the *Journal of the American Medical Association* (JAMA). The analysis includes those with hemorrhagic and nonhemorrhagic presentation. The quote is from the article. AVM, arteriovenous malformation. (*Data from* van Beijnum J, van der Worp HB, Buis DR, et al. Treatment of brain arteriovenous malformations: a systematic review and meta-analysis. JAMA 2011;306:2011; with permission.)

"perfusion–pressure breakthrough" after feeding artery occlusion.[48] This latter issue was subsequently found to be related to cerebral hyperemia, but not to feeding artery pressure.[49] Initial efforts at embolization used small pellets of Silastic impregnated with barium and fragments of muscle removed from the adjacent sternocleidomastoid muscle, directly injected into the feeding arteries during open surgery.[50] The field rapidly developed toward transfemoral catheters delivering a variety of embolic materials, ranging from polyvinyl alcohol,[51] low-viscosity silicone rubber,[52] prothrombotic metal, N-butyl cyanoacrylate glues,[53] and more recently ethylene vinyl alcohol (Onyx).[54] None of these agents are free of risk, especially when the material deposits in the venous outflow before complete occlusion of the bAVM.[55] Guglielmi detachable coils are among the devices used.[56] Despite large cohorts from single centers, most reports do not cite outcomes for those not having bled before intervention,[17] but some of the most recent have done so, noting nonhemorrhagic presentation as predictor for new deficits (P<.002).[57]

Not to be denied, radiotherapy has also provided a large experience[58] and, as with the other modalities, with widely varying results.[59] Radiotherapy is becoming increasingly popular, given its apparent noninvasive qualities. Its use has been shown to obliterate some of the smaller lesions.[60] Higher doses were required for the larger lesions, with uncertainty of success and concern for radiation necrosis.[61,62] Minakawa and colleagues[10] repeated the angiogram 5 to 28 years after first discovery or treatment in 20 patients, 16 of whom were untreated; the remaining were residual. The AVM was unchanged in 8, larger in 4, smaller in 4, and had disappeared in 4. The AVMs that disappeared were relatively small and fed by a single feeder or a few feeders. Meta-analyses have shown a wide range of outcomes, not segregated by nonhemorrhagic presentation.[15] A recent report of late follow-up from some centers has documented a rate for those with nonhemorrhagic presentation of 1.2% compared with 3.3% for those hemorrhagic.[63]

Treatments may fall short of total obliteration of the AVM owing to halt of the program.

Once an AVM has been removed (as proved by postoperative angiography), recurrent hemorrhage presumably should not occur, but recurrence has been documented in a small portion of the literature.[64] There is no useful literature on the long-term outcome for those with incomplete removal of the bAVM.[23,24]

THE UNRUPTURED BRAIN ARTERIOVENOUS MALFORMATIONS TRIAL

A randomised trial, Unruptured Brain Arteriovenous malformations (ARUBA), funded by the National Institute of Neurological Disorders and Stroke (NINDS), was reported recently.[65] It was designed to establish whether, for those with a bAVM discovered not to have bled, the long-term outcomes for medical management were comparable, inferior, or superior to "interventional therapy." The interventions were those in common practice, namely, endovascular procedures, neurosurgery, or radiotherapy, and could be used alone or in any combination. The interventional arm was considered the "standard therapy," and while the medical arm was the "experimental" arm.

The trail was funded by the NINDS in 2006; 66 centers world-wide agreed to participate. The trial recruited 226 patients from 39 active centers world-wide at a steady rate of 3 per month beginning in April 2007. At a preplanned meeting with investigators April 2013, the NINDS-selected Data Safety Monitoring Board (DSMB) recommended cessation of randomizations. This recommendation was based on their review of a preplanned interim analysis that revealed patients assigned to receive interventional therapy were more than 3 times more likely to experience a stroke or death during the follow-up period than their counterparts (33 months on average; hazard ratio, 3.41; 95% CI, 1.72–6.76). When randomization was halted, 48% of the cohort were entirely asymptomatic, 62% had a bAVM of less than 3 cm, 66% had superficial drainage, and 100% had a modified Rankin score of 0 or 1 (48% were zero; **Fig. 2**).

The DSMB also recommended further follow-up for all participants to determine whether the disparities in stroke and death rates would change. The follow-up would assess whether such differences translated into a clinically meaningful difference in long-term functional outcome. These points were the basis for the formal NINDS announcement, posted on their website on May 9, 2013 (http://www.ninds.nih.gov/news_and_events/news_articles/ARUBA_trial_results.htm). The results were presented at the 23rd annual European Stroke Conference (London, UK) and published in Lancet (Epub November 2013 with formal publication February 2014).[66] Its major finding favored the medical arm in the analysis "as randomized" and even more "as treated" (**Fig. 3**).

Criticisms of the Unruptured Brain Arteriovenous Malformations Trial and Responses

During the active phase of ARUBA, a steady stream of criticisms was published[67,68] and rebutted.[69,70] After publication, more criticisms appeared.[71–73] Many criticisms were based on undocumented inferences of biased patient selection, low skills from participating centers, low participation from alleged major centers, uncommon choices for intervention, low enrollment compared with those screened, and lack of reporting on outcomes from those eligible but not randomized. Each of the major criticisms has received public presentation or published response: The demographics of the population match those reported from defined major populations[69]; the distribution of Spetzler–Martin grades was indeed biased, but toward the more easily

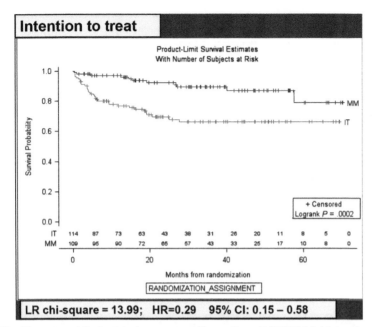

Fig. 2. The Unruptured Brain Arteriovenous malformations (ARUBA) trial intention-to-treat analysis showing superiority of the medical arm.

treated[74]; and the participating centers showed their qualifications by more than 600 publications found in PubMed for the years 2000 to 2010. The choices for intervention correspond with those most often published from individual centers. The criticism that too few underwent surgery only[75] is rebutted by the lack of reference to surgery as a single treatment modality in the only management algorithm published for those not having bled.[76] Surgery was a treatment plan for 21 of the 100 patients (**Fig. 4**). The fate of those eligible but not randomized remains unreported because no participating center responded to the offer of a registry for such patients. The widely claimed 4% participation implies that more than 1400 screened patients were all eligible, but all but 500 were ineligible owing to prior hemorrhage or intervention, and the for those eligible among the 39 active centers the randomization rate was fully 61%. Criticisms of the lack of data on microhemorrhages in assessment of unbled bAVMs[77] cannot be answered because the 2012 date of publication on microhemorrhages as a risk factor for rupture precluded its inclusion in the formal protocol during the trial. Finally, the brief mean time of follow-up was the result of the halting of the randomization phase by the DSMB, not the plan of the investigators. However, based on the disparity in outcome events between the 2 arms in the trial, study statisticians calculated a range of 12 to 30 years might be needed for events in the medical arm to reach that of the intervention group, assuming no further events occur in the intervention group.[78] We offer no comment on a recent complaint that neurosurgeons are being referred fewer cases for neurovascular surgery, and for the inference that the large number of cases eligible but treated outside for a trial presumably had satisfactory results.[79]

Subset Results

Reluctant to report data from small subsets in our trial, we have recently responded to postpublication criticism that the reported stroke outcomes in the interventional arm

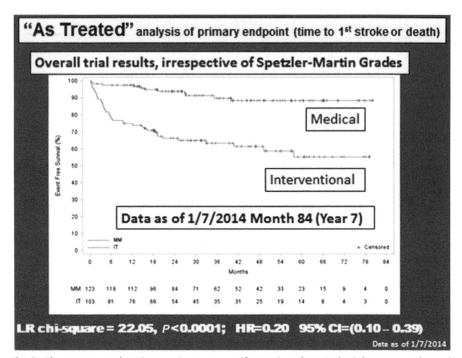

"As Treated" analysis of primary endpoint (time to 1st stroke or death)

Overall trial results, irrespective of Spetzler-Martin Grades

Medical

Interventional

Data as of 1/7/2014 Month 84 (Year 7)

LR chi-square = 22.05, $P < 0.0001$; HR=0.20 95% CI=(0.10 – 0.39)

Data as of 1/7/2014

Fig. 3. The Unruptured Brain Arteriovenous malformations (ARUBA) trial "as-treated" analysis. Those randomized to the medical arm who crossed over to the intervention arm and experienced an event from intervention are counted in the intervention arm; those randomized to the intervention arm who had an outcome event before initiation of the intervention are counted in the medical arm.

might contain a large number of clinically minor events, for example, headache with a positive MR. Such events would have been counted as stroke because a new symptom was associated with a new infarct or hemorrhage documented by MR (ARUBA clinical protocol).[66] We agree a clear statement is needed on the functional effect of stroke outcomes. Analysis of the modified Rankin score status at the time of the outcome event showed a modified Rankin score of 2 or more for only 2 of the 8 in the medical arm, but for 28 of 34 in the interventional arm.[74] Recalculation of the odds ratio between the 2 arms of the trial showed a further favorable shift in the direction of the medical arm in the "as treated" when the outcomes were limited to those with modified Rankin score of 2 or greater.

THE FUTURE

The current status of the data from ARUBA leaves unsettled both the long-term rate of hemorrhage and hemorrhage severity for those in the medical arm. The investigators, backed by the DSMB and the NINDS Clinical Notice, applied for continued follow-up of the ARUBA cohort, but were denied funding. Among the comments from reviewers was the inference that the data would change little in the coming 5 years.

A unique opportunity still exists to clarify the long-term risk and the severity of hemorrhage in this well-characterized cohort of unbled bAVMs. The ARUBA study contains 500 cases eligible for the trial. All of them, randomized or not, are well-characterized, known to ARUBA centers, and presumably available for follow-up.

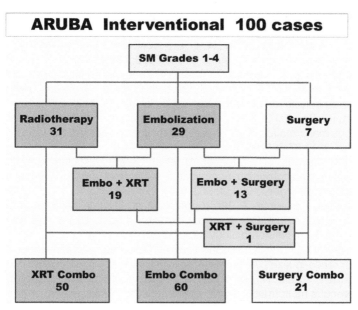

Fig. 4. Interventional management for the 100 randomized to the intervention arm in the Unruptured Brain Arteriovenous malformations (ARUBA) trial. Embo, embolization; XRT, radiotherapy.

Many active centers are continuing to contribute follow-up for randomized cases pro bono. Their access to their patients could also permit assessment of those newly described potential risk factors for hemorrhage: silent intralesional microhemorrhage[77] and single draining vein status.[80] An update of cost factors for invasive management could also be included.[81]

The resultant data would be a modern epidemiologic documentation of the prevalence of bAVMs and incidence data for adverse outcomes for several well-characterized populations. The emphasis on those discovered to be unbled would provide a benchmark against which presumable improvements in interventions for lesion eradication could be compared.

CLINICALLY EFFICACY OF THERAPEUTIC INTERVENTIONS

In adult patients ($\geq$18 years) with an unruptured bAVM, addition of interventional therapy (ie, neurosurgery, embolization, or stereotactic radiotherapy, alone or in combination) to medical management alone (ie, pharmacologic therapy for neurologic symptoms as needed) is probably harmful (level of clinical efficacy, 2-X; level of evidence, T1).

REFERENCES

1. Perret G, Nishioka H. Report on the cooperative study of intracranial aneurysms and subarachnoid hemorrhage. Section VI. Arteriovenous malformations. An analysis of 545 cases of cranio-cerebral arteriovenous malformations and fistulae reported to the cooperative study. J Neurosurg 1966;25:467–90.
2. Gross CR, Kase CS, Mohr JP, et al. Stroke in south Alabama: incidence and diagnostic features–a population based study. Stroke 1984;15:249–55.

3. McCormick WF. The pathology of vascular ("arteriovenous") malformations. J Neurosurg 1966;24:807–16.
4. Stapf C, Mast H, Sciacca RR, et al. The New York Islands AVM Study: design, study progress, and initial results. Stroke 2003;34:e29–33.
5. Al-Shahi R, Fang JS, Lewis SC, et al. Prevalence of adults with brain arteriovenous malformations: a community based study in Scotland using capture-recapture analysis. J Neurol Neurosurg Psychiatry 2002;73:547–51.
6. Kilbourn KJ, Spiegel G, Killory BD, et al. Case report of a de novo brainstem arteriovenous malformation in an 18-year-old male and review of the literature. Neurosurg Rev 2014;37:685–91.
7. Batjer HH, Devous MD Sr, Meyer YJ, et al. Cerebrovascular hemodynamics in arteriovenous malformation complicated by normal perfusion pressure breakthrough. Neurosurgery 1988;22:503–9.
8. Willinsky RA, Lasjaunias P, Terbrugge K, et al. Multiple cerebral arteriovenous malformations (AVMs). Review of our experience from 203 patients with cerebral vascular lesions. Neuroradiology 1990;32:207–10.
9. Mendelow AD, Erfurth A, Grossart K, et al. Do cerebral arteriovenous malformations increase in size? J Neurol Neurosurg Psychiatry 1987;50:980–7.
10. Minakawa T, Tanaka R, Koike T, et al. Angiographic follow-up study of cerebral arteriovenous malformations with reference to their enlargement and regression. Neurosurgery 1989;24:68–74.
11. Stein BM, Wolpert SM. Arteriovenous malformations of the brain. I: current concepts and treatment. Arch Neurol 1980;37:1–5.
12. Jane J, Kassell NF, Torner JC, et al. The natural history of aneurysms and arteriovenous malformations. J Neurosurg 1985;62:321.
13. Crawford P, West CR, Chadwick DW, et al. Arteriovenous malformations of the brain: natural history in unoperated patients. J Neurol Neurosurg Psychiatry 1986;49:1.
14. Ondra SL, Troupp H, George ED, et al. The natural history of symptomatic arteriovenous malformations of the brain: a 24-year follow-up assessment. J Neurosurg 1990;73:387–91.
15. van Beijnum J, van der Worp HB, Buis DR, et al. Treatment of brain arteriovenous malformations: a systematic review and meta-analysis. JAMA 2011;306:2011–9.
16. Lawton MT, Du R, Tran MN, et al. Effect of presenting hemorrhage on outcome after microsurgical resection of brain arteriovenous malformations. Neurosurgery 2005;56:485–93 [discussion: 485–93].
17. Jayaraman MV, Marcellus ML, Hamilton S, et al. Neurologic complications of arteriovenous malformation embolization using liquid embolic agents. AJNR Am J Neuroradiol 2008;29:242–6.
18. Maruyama K, Kawahara N, Shin M, et al. The risk of hemorrhage after radiosurgery for cerebral arteriovenous malformations. N Engl J Med 2005;352:146–53.
19. Stapf C, Mohr JP, Choi JH, et al. Invasive treatment of unruptured brain arteriovenous malformations is experimental therapy. Curr Opin Neurol 2006;19:63–8.
20. Hillman J. Population-based analysis of arteriovenous malformation treatment. J Neurosurg 2001;95:633–7.
21. ApSimon HT, Reef H, Phadke RV, et al. A population-based study of brain arteriovenous malformation: long-term treatment outcomes. Stroke 2002;33:2794–800.
22. Hartmann A, Mast H, Choi JH, et al. Treatment of arteriovenous malformations of the brain. Curr Neurol Neurosci Rep 2007;7:28–34.
23. Stapf C, Mohr JP, Pile-Spellman J, et al. Epidemiology and natural history of arteriovenous malformations. Neurosurg Focus 2001;11:e1.

24. Al-Shahi R, Bhattacharya JJ, Currie DG, et al. Prospective, population-based detection of intracranial vascular malformations in adults: the Scottish Intracranial Vascular Malformation Study (SIVMS). Stroke 2003;34:1163–9.
25. Brown RD Jr, Wiebers DO, Forbes GS. Unruptured intracranial aneurysms and arteriovenous malformations: frequency of intracranial hemorrhage and relationship of lesions. J Neurosurg 1990;73:859–63.
26. Brown RD Jr, Wiebers DO, Forbes G, et al. The natural history of unruptured intracranial arteriovenous malformations. J Neurosurg 1988;68:352–7.
27. Abecassis IJ, Xu DS, Batjer HH, et al. Natural history of brain arteriovenous malformations: a systematic review. Neurosurg Focus 2014;37:E7.
28. Stapf C, Mohr JP, Sciacca RR, et al. Incident hemorrhage risk of brain arteriovenous malformations located in the arterial border zones. Stroke 2000;31:2365–8.
29. Choi JH, Mohr JP. Brain arteriovenous malformations in adults. Lancet Neurol 2005;4:299–308.
30. Hartmann A, Mast H, Mohr JP, et al. Morbidity of intracranial hemorrhage in patients with cerebral arteriovenous malformation. Stroke 1998;29:931–4.
31. Lobato RD, Gomez PA, Rivas JJ. Arteriovenous malformations and vasospasm. J Neurosurg 1998;88:934–5.
32. N DWC. Angiomatous malformations of the brain. Guys Hosp Rep 1940;90:149.
33. Mackenzie I. The clinical presentation of the cerebral angioma; a review of 50 cases. Brain 1953;76:184–214.
34. Lees F. The migrainous symptoms of cerebral angiomata. J Neurol Neurosurg Psychiatry 1962;25:45.
35. Haas DC. Arteriovenous malformations and migraine: case reports and an analysis of the relationship. Headache 1991;31:509–13.
36. Galletti F, Sarchielli P, Hamam M, et al. Occipital arteriovenous malformations and migraine. Cephalalgia 2011;31:1320–4.
37. Garcin B, Houdart E, Porcher R, et al. Epileptic seizures at initial presentation in patients with brain arteriovenous malformation. Neurology 2012;78:626–31.
38. Josephson CB, Leach JP, Duncan R, et al. Seizure risk from cavernous or arteriovenous malformations: prospective population-based study. Neurology 2011;76:1548–54.
39. Al-Shahi Salman R, White PM, Counsell CE, et al. Outcome after conservative management or intervention for unruptured brain arteriovenous malformations. JAMA 2014;311:1661–9.
40. Nornes H, Grip A. Hemodynamic aspects of cerebral arteriovenous malformations. J Neurosurg 1980;53:456–64.
41. Mast H, Mohr JP, Osipov A, et al. 'Steal' is an unestablished mechanism for the clinical presentation of cerebral arteriovenous malformations. Stroke 1995;26:1215–20.
42. Carter LP, Gumerlock MK. Steal and cerebral arteriovenous malformations. Stroke 1995;26:2371–2.
43. Racine CA, Lawton MT, Hetts SW, et al. Neuropyschological profile of reversible cognitive impairment in a patient with a dural arteriovenous fistula. Neurocase 2008;14:231–8.
44. Choi JH, Mast H, Hartmann A, et al. Clinical and morphological determinants of focal neurological deficits in patients with unruptured brain arteriovenous malformation. J Neurol Sci 2009;287:126–30.
45. Steiger HJ, Etminan N, Hanggi D. Epilepsy and headache after resection of cerebral arteriovenous malformations. Acta Neurochir Suppl 2014;119:113–5.
46. Spetzler RF, Martin NA. A proposed grading system for arteriovenous malformations. J Neurosurg 1986;65:476–83.

47. Kim H, Abla AA, Nelson J, et al. Validation of the supplemented Spetzler-Martin grading system for brain arteriovenous malformations in a multicenter cohort of 1009 surgical patients. Neurosurgery 2015;76:25–33.
48. Spetzler RF, Wilson CB, Weinstein P, et al. Normal perfusion pressure breakthrough theory. Clin Neurosurg 1978;25:651–72.
49. Young WL, Kader A, Ornstein E, et al. Cerebral hyperemia after arteriovenous malformation resection is related to "breakthrough" complications but not to feeding artery pressure. The Columbia University Arteriovenous Malformation Study Project. Neurosurgery 1996;38:1085–93 [discussion: 1093–5].
50. Luessenhop AJ, Mujica PH. Embolization of segments of the circle of Willis and adjacent branches for management of certain inoperable cerebral arteriovenous malformations. J Neurosurg 1981;54:573–82.
51. Sorimachi T, Koike T, Takeuchi S, et al. Embolization of cerebral arteriovenous malformations achieved with polyvinyl alcohol particles: angiographic reappearance and complications. AJNR Am J Neuroradiol 1999;20:1323–8.
52. Hilal SK, Sane P, Michelson WJ, et al. The embolization of vascular malformations of the spinal cord with low-viscosity silicone rubber. Neuroradiology 1978;16:430–3.
53. DeMeritt JS, Pile-Spellman J, Mast H, et al. Outcome analysis of preoperative embolization with N-butyl cyanoacrylate in cerebral arteriovenous malformations. AJNR Am J Neuroradiol 1995;16:1801–7.
54. Sanborn MR, Park MS, McDougall CG, et al. Endovascular approaches to pial arteriovenous malformations. Neurosurg Clin N Am 2014;25:529–37.
55. Baharvahdat H, Blanc R, Termechi R, et al. Hemorrhagic complications after endovascular treatment of cerebral arteriovenous malformations. AJNR Am J Neuroradiol 2014;35:978–83.
56. Luo CB, Teng MM, Chang FC, et al. Endovascular treatment of intracranial high-flow arteriovenous fistulas by Guglielmi detachable coils. J Chin Med Assoc 2006;69:80–5.
57. Pandey P, Marks MP, Harraher CD, et al. Multimodality management of Spetzler-Martin Grade III arteriovenous malformations. J Neurosurg 2012;116:1279–88.
58. Bendok BR, El Tecle NE, El Ahmadieh TY, et al. Advances and innovations in brain arteriovenous malformation surgery. Neurosurgery 2014;74(Suppl 1):S60–73.
59. van Beijnum J, Bhattacharya JJ, Counsell CE, et al. Patterns of brain arteriovenous malformation treatment: prospective, population-based study. Stroke 2008;39:3216–21.
60. Candia GJ, Kjellberg RN, Lyons S. Proton-beam therapy for cerebral arteriovenous-malformations. J Neurosurg 1990;72:A334.
61. Bostrom J, Hadizadeh DR, Block W, et al. Magnetic resonance spectroscopic study of radiogenic changes after radiosurgery of cerebral arteriovenous malformations with implications for the differential diagnosis of radionecrosis. Radiat Oncol 2013;8:54.
62. Parkhutik V, Lago A, Aparici F, et al. Late clinical and radiological complications of stereotactical radiosurgery of arteriovenous malformations of the brain. Neuroradiology 2013;55:405–12.
63. Parkhutik V, Lago A, Tembl JI, et al. Postradiosurgery hemorrhage rates of arteriovenous malformations of the brain influencing factors and evolution with time. Stroke 2012;43:1247–52.
64. Hashimoto N, Nozaki K. Do cerebral arteriovenous malformations recur after angiographically confirmed total extirpation? Crit Rev Neurosurg 1999;9:141–6.

65. Mohr JP. A randomized trial of unruptured brain arteriovenous malformations (ARUBA). Acta Neurochir Suppl 2008;103:3–4.
66. Mohr JP, Parides MK, Stapf C, et al. Medical management with or without interventional therapy for unruptured brain arteriovenous malformations (ARUBA): a multicentre, non-blinded, randomised trial. Lancet 2014;383:614–21.
67. Cockroft KM. Unruptured cerebral arteriovenous malformations: to treat or not to treat. Stroke 2006;37:1148–9.
68. Cockroft KM, Jayaraman MV, Amin-Hanjani S, et al. A perfect storm: how a randomized trial of unruptured brain arteriovenous malformations' (ARUBA's) trial design challenges notions of external validity. Stroke 2012;43:1979–81.
69. Mohr JP, Moskowitz AJ, Stapf C, et al. The ARUBA trial: current status, future hopes. Stroke 2010;41:e537–40.
70. Mohr JP, Moskowitz AJ, Parides M, et al. Hull down on the horizon: A Randomized trial of Unruptured Brain Arteriovenous malformations (ARUBA) trial. Stroke 2012; 43:1744–5.
71. Bambakidis NC, Cockroft K, Connolly ES, et al. Preliminary results of the ARUBA study. Neurosurgery 2013;73:E379–81.
72. Solomon RA, Connolly ES Jr. Management of brain arteriovenous malformations. Lancet 2014;383:1634.
73. Amin-Hanjani S, Albuquerque FC, Britz G, et al. Commentary: unruptured brain arteriovenous malformations: what a tangled web they weave. Neurosurgery 2014;75:195–6.
74. Mohr JP. Results of ARUBA are applicable to most patients with nonruptured arteriovenous malformations. Stroke 2014;45:1541–2.
75. Stapf C, Parides MK, Moskowitz AJ, et al. Management of brain arteriovenous malformations–authors' reply. Lancet 2014;383:1635–6.
76. Steig PE, Batjer HH, Samson D. Intracranial arteriovenous malformations. New York: Informa; 2007.
77. Guo Y, Saunders T, Su H, et al. Silent intralesional microhemorrhage as a risk factor for brain arteriovenous malformation rupture. Stroke 2012;43:1240–6.
78. Parides MK, Overbey JR, Stapf C, et al. Projecting longer term results in the ARUBA trial. 2014; Session 5 Large Clinical Trials, 23rd European Stroke Conference. Nice, France, May 9, 2014.
79. Korja M, Hernesniemi J, Lawton MT, et al. Is cerebrovascular neurosurgery sacrificed on the altar of RCTs? Lancet 2014;384:27–8.
80. Sahlein DH, Mora P, Becske T, et al. Features predictive of brain arteriovenous malformation hemorrhage: extrapolation to a physiologic model. Stroke 2014; 45:1964–70.
81. Berman MF, Hartmann A, Mast H, et al. Determinants of resource utilization in the treatment of brain arteriovenous malformations. AJNR Am J Neuroradiol 1999;20: 2004–8.

Acute Treatment of Blood Pressure After Ischemic Stroke and Intracerebral Hemorrhage

J. Dedrick Jordan, MD, PhD[a,b,]*, Kathryn A. Morbitzer, PharmD[c],
Denise H. Rhoney, PharmD, FNCS[c]

KEYWORDS

- Acute ischemic stroke • Intracerebral hemorrhage • Blood pressure
- Hemorrhagic conversion • Hematoma expansion • Cerebral edema • Hypertension

KEY POINTS

- Aggressive blood pressure (BP) reduction in patients with acute ischemic stroke who do not qualify for thrombolysis has not been shown to improve outcomes.
- For patients who qualify for intravenous thrombolysis with alteplase, BP elevated more than 185/110 mm Hg before initiation of thrombolytic therapy or 180/105 mm Hg during the 24 hours after treatment has been associated with worse clinical outcomes.
- BP variability seems to be linked to poor functional outcomes and increased risk of hemorrhagic transformation of cerebral infarction.
- Aggressive BP reduction in patients with intracerebral hemorrhage does not cause significant cerebral hypoperfusion and ischemia in the perihematomal region.
- Aggressive BP reduction is safe in patients with intracerebral hemorrhage but has been shown to not significantly improve clinical outcomes.

ISCHEMIC STROKE

Management of the early elevation in blood pressure (BP) following acute ischemic stroke (AIS) is a major unresolved issue in current clinical management. Although it may seem logical to decrease BP acutely with antihypertensive medications, there

[a] Department of Neurology, University of North Carolina at Chapel Hill School of Medicine, 2118 Physician Office Building, Campus Box 7025, Chapel Hill, NC 27599, USA; [b] Department of Neurosurgery, University of North Carolina at Chapel Hill School of Medicine, 2118 Physician Office Building, Campus Box 7025, Chapel Hill, NC 27599, USA; [c] Division of Practice Advancement and Clinical Education, UNC Eshelman School of Pharmacy, University of North Carolina at Chapel Hill, 115 Beard Hall, Campus Box 7574, Chapel Hill, NC 27599, USA
* Corresponding author.
E-mail address: dedrick@unc.edu

Neurol Clin 33 (2015) 361–380
http://dx.doi.org/10.1016/j.ncl.2014.12.003 **neurologic.theclinics.com**
0733-8619/15/$ – see front matter © 2015 Elsevier Inc. All rights reserved.

are reasonable arguments physiologically to support both lowering BP and refraining from early BP reduction (permissive hypertension). The rationale for lowering BP is to reduce or prevent cerebral edema and limit hemorrhagic transformation of the infarct. Alternatively, the concern with lowering BP in AIS is the expansion of the central ischemic core by worsening hypoperfusion within the ischemic penumbra, because this area may have disrupted cerebral autoregulation. The key clinical questions that are reviewed based on the currently available evidence include the following: (1) When should antihypertensive therapy be started following AIS? (2) How fast and what goal BP should be targeted? (3) Which is the best antihypertensive agent to use in AIS?

Abnormal Blood Pressure in Acute Ischemic Stroke

Many patients with AIS will present to the emergency department with hypertension; however, it is unclear whether this represents a natural compensatory mechanism or is related to a wide array of other causes, such as pain, dehydration, or chronic illness.[1,2] Several studies have been helpful in describing the natural history of BP changes following AIS (**Table 1**).

Two large multicenter trials, the Chinese Acute Stroke Trial (CAST) with 21,106 patients and the International Stroke Trial (IST) with 19,435 patients, were originally designed to assess antiplatelet use in AIS; however, these trials also produced significant information regarding hypertension in the acute phase following ischemic stroke.[3,4] CAST reported hypertension (defined as systolic BP [SBP] greater than 140 mm Hg) in 75% of patients with an acute stroke within the first 2 days, whereas the IST reported the incidence as 80%. Marked hypertension (defined as SBP >180 mm Hg) was seen in 25% of patients in CAST and 28% of patients in IST. The findings of CAST and IST have been supported by a large observational trial. Qureshi and colleagues[5] evaluated the prevalence of elevated BP using a large data set comprising 276,734 patients presenting to the emergency department with AIS. An SBP of 140 mm Hg or greater was observed in 76.5% of patients based on their initial measurement.

Although not universal, the natural history of hypertension postischemic stroke has seemed to involve an initial acute increase, followed by a reduction over the next several days.[1,2,6,7] The Barcelona Downtown stroke registry found that an early decrease of SBP by 20% to 30% was associated with a full recovery.[8] In patients treated with intra-arterial thrombolysis, decreases in SBP early after AIS have been associated with recanalization of the vessel.[9]

Recently, findings have suggested that for BP measured within 3 hours of stroke onset, the mean first SBP is only slightly higher than the premorbid level (a 17.9 mm Hg increase vs most recent SBP and a 10.6 mm Hg increase vs 10-year mean premorbid level).[10] This finding contrasts with the significant increase in BP compared with premorbid levels in intracerebral hemorrhage (ICH), which may provide reasoning behind the differences seen in the risks and benefits of lowering BP acutely after stroke.

Cerebral Autoregulation in Acute Ischemic Stroke

Under normal conditions, cerebral blood flow is maintained within a tight range despite variation in systemic pressure. This equilibrium is achieved through cerebral autoregulation (**Fig. 1**).[11] The dynamic cerebral vasculature either constricts or dilates in response to changes in mean arterial pressure (MAP) ranging from 50 to 150 mm Hg in order to maintain a stable cerebral blood flow.[12,13] On the lower end of this zone of autoregulation, cerebral ischemia eventually occurs when the pressure remains less than the lower limit of autoregulation. Conversely, cerebral vessels constrict as

MAP increases and the vascular endothelial cells become stretched. Eventually, the cerebral vessels can no longer constrict effectively against the high perfusion pressure and autoregulation fails, which may lead to cerebral edema or hemorrhage. Chronic untreated hypertension may impact autoregulation whereby the zone of autoregulation is shifted to the right toward higher pressures. Cerebral autoregulation may be impaired following AIS as cerebral blood flow more closely reflects the systemic arterial BP, although this is controversial with inconsistent data from human and animal studies.[14] Therefore, hypertension following an AIS may reflect a compensatory or protective physiologic response aimed at maintaining perfusion of the ischemic penumbra.[13,15]

If the hypertensive response is protective it raises the clinical controversy as to if and when acute hypertension should be treated following AIS. Increased BP raises concern for secondary complications, such as hemorrhagic transformation and exacerbating cerebral edema.[16,17] However, if cerebral autoregulation is not maintained, then lowering the BP acutely could worsen hypoperfusion within the penumbra.[13] This clinical response provides theoretic reasoning behind maintaining or raising the BP during the acute period following AIS.

Blood Pressure as a Prognostic Indicator in Acute Ischemic Stroke

The optimal targets for BP management in patients with AIS remain uncertain, as several observational studies have demonstrated a U-shaped correlation with poor outcomes. In these studies, poor outcomes were seen with either very high or very low admission BP.

Baseline BP data from the IST were analyzed to explore the relationship between SBP and clinical events and functional outcomes. In evaluating greater than 17,000 patients with confirmed ischemic stroke, the investigators found that both high BP and low BP were independent prognostic indicators for poor outcomes (death within 14 days or death or dependency at 6 months). A baseline SBP of 140 to 179 mm Hg, with the nadir at 150 mm Hg, resulted in the lowest frequency of poor outcomes.[18] A prospective observational study comprising greater than 900 patients with AIS also demonstrated early and late mortality in relation to a U-shaped curve admission SBP pattern. Vemmos and colleagues[19] found that the relative risk of 1-month and 1-year mortality increased with a 10-mm Hg SBP change greater than or less than 130 mm Hg. Although both of these studies demonstrated an association with poor outcomes and a U-shaped SBP curve, the reference point for the ideal SBP differs, resulting in an unclear prognostic indicator.

Other studies have found associations between one direction of SBP and patient outcomes. In a cohort of 357 patients with AIS, Stead and colleagues[20] found that patients with SBP less than 155 mm Hg were more likely to die within 90 days than patients presenting with an SBP between 155 and 220 mm Hg. Alternatively, 265 patients with AIS were analyzed in the Intravenous Nimodipine West European Stroke Trial and found differing results. The study defined high initial BP as an initial BP greater than 160/90 mm Hg. They found that high initial BP was a predictor for death or dependency at 21 days compared with patients who had a normal initial BP (SBP 120–160 mm Hg and diastolic BP 60–90 mm Hg).[21] Conversely, Jensen and colleagues[22] found that although a higher initial SBP reduced the odds of a good outcome, after adjusting for other prognostic indicators, it was not an independent predictor of a good outcome. This finding suggests that hypertension on admission may be a marker of other factors, such as the severity of the stroke or a sign of premorbid hypertension, rather than an independent prognostic guide.

A limitation of these studies is the use of only admission BP in making these outcome assessments. An analysis of the Virtual Stroke International Stroke Trial

Table 1
Key trials evaluating BP control in acute stroke

Trial	Design	Study Arms/Cohort	Number of Patients	Time from Onset to Presentation	Results
AIS					
CATIS[30]	Randomized, single-blind, blinded end point, prospective	Antihypertensive treatment vs discontinue all antihypertensive medications	4071	<48 h	No difference seen in death or major disability at hospital discharge or 2 wk or at 3 mo
VISTA Collaboration[23]	Academic collaboration with data obtained from randomized trials	Patients with hyperacute IS who received placebo treatment	1722	<8 h	High SBP and large variability in SBP in hyperacute stages of IS are associated with increased neurologic impairment and poor functional outcome
Fukuoka Stroke Registry[24]	Multicenter, prospective stroke registry	First-ever AIS who had been functionally independent before onset	1874	<24 h	SBP range of 144–153 mm Hg and greater associated with lower probability of good neurologic recovery
AIS-Thrombolysis					
SITS-ISTR[40]	Retrospective analysis of prospectively collected register	Hypertensive patients treated with antihypertensives vs hypertensive patients and withholding antihypertensives vs patients without history of hypertension and treated with hypertensives vs patients without history of hypertension and not treated with antihypertensives	11,080	Median (IQR) 145 h (115–170)	Increased SBP 2–24 h after thrombolytic therapy associated with worse outcomes at 3 mo. Best outcomes observed with SBP between 141–150 mm Hg after thrombolysis
SAMURAI rt-PA Registry[45]	Retrospective, observational	Patients with AIS who received IV rt-PA	527	Median (IQR) 141 min (121–165)	Early SBP variability positively associated with ICH and death

	Study design	Intervention	N	Time	Outcome
AIS/ICH					
CHHIPS[28]	Randomized, double-blinded, prospective	Labetalol vs lisinopril vs placebo	179	<36 h	No difference in death or dependency at 2 wk; In active treatment arm, 3-mo mortality was reduced
SCAST[29]	Randomized, double-blinded, prospective	Candesartan vs placebo	2004	<30 h	Trend toward increased risk of poor functional outcomes at 6 mo in candesartan group
COSSACS[31]	Open, blinded end point, prospective	Continue vs discontinue preexisting antihypertensive drug	763	<48 h	No difference observed in death or dependency at 2 wk
ENOS[32]	Randomized, single-blinded, blinded-outcome, prospective	Glyceryl trinitrate vs continuing premorbid antihypertensive therapy vs discontinuing antihypertensive medications	4000	<48 h	No difference found in modified Rankin score at 90 d between continuing vs stopping premorbid antihypertensive therapy
Liu-DeRyke et al,[34] 2008	Pseudorandomized, prospective	Labetalol vs nicardipine	54	—	Patients in nicardipine group achieved higher rate of goal BP within 60 min, had better maintenance of BP, had greater percentage of time spent within goal BP range, and had less BP variability
ICH					
INTERACT[73]	Randomized, blinded-outcome, prospective	Intensive- (SBP <140 mm Hg) vs guideline- (SBP <180 mm Hg) based BP control	346	<6 h	Early intensive BP reduction is feasible and may reduce hematoma expansion
ATACH[74]	Dose escalation, prospective	SBP 170–200 mm Hg vs SBP 140–170 mm Hg vs 110–140 mm Hg	60	<6 h	Early intensive BP reduction is safe and feasible
INTERACT2[77]	Randomized, open-treatment, blinded-outcome, prospective	SBP <140 mm Hg vs SBP <180 mm Hg	2839	<6 h	No difference found in modified Rankin score at 90 d

Abbreviations: ATACH, Antihypertensive Treatment of Acute Cerebral Hemorrhage; CATIS, Chinese Antihypertensive Trial in Acute Ischemic Stroke; CHHIPS, Controlling Hypertension and Hypotension Immediately Post-Stroke; COSSACS, Continue Or Stop post-Stroke Antihypertensives Collaborative Study; ENOS, Efficacy of Nitric Oxide in Stroke; ICH, intracerebral hemorrhage; INTERACT, Intensive Blood Pressure Reduction in Acute Cerebral Hemorrhage Trial; IQR, interquartile range; IS, ischemic stroke; IV, intravenous; rt-PA, recombinant tissue plasminogen activator; SAMURAI, Stroke Acute Management With Urgent Risk-factor Assessment and Improvement; SBP, systolic BP; SITS-ISTR, Safe Implementation of Thrombolysis in Stroke–International Stroke Thrombolysis Register; SCAST, The Angiotensin-Receptor Blocker Candesartan for Treatment of Acute Stroke; VISTA, Virtual Stroke International Stroke Trial Archive.

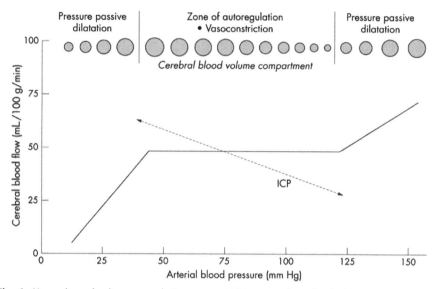

Fig. 1. Normal cerebral autoregulation curve. With normal cerebral physiology, the brain maintains a stable cerebral blood flow (CBF) under a wide range of mean arterial pressure (MAPs) (range: 50–150 mm Hg). When MAP decreases less than or exceeds the limit of autoregulation, CBF becomes pressure dependent. (*From* Lang EW, Lagopoulos J, Griffith J, et al. Cerebral vasomotor reactivity testing in head injury: the link between pressure and flow. J Neurol Neurosurg Psychiatr 2003;74(8):1053–9; with permission.)

Archive (VISTA) collaboration examined the relationship between hemodynamic measures, variability in BP, and change in BP over the first 24 hours after AIS.[23] High SBP measured initially and with subsequent measurement up to 24 hours was significantly associated with increased neurologic impairment and poor functional outcomes. The magnitude of change in BP over this first 24 hours was also significantly related to poor outcomes whereby patients having large decreases in BP (>75 mm Hg) or increases (>25 mm Hg) seemed to have the highest risk of poor outcomes.[23]

Recognizing the controversy surrounding the association between postischemic stroke BP and patient outcomes, Ishitsuka and colleagues[24] developed a large-scale stroke registry aimed at assessing this relationship. Analysis of the registry showed that the SBP (averaged over first 48 hours) range of 144 to 153 mm Hg and greater was associated with a lower probability of good neurologic recovery, even after multiple adjustments for potential confounders. Similar relationships were found in that higher SBP was also associated with elevated risks of neurologic deterioration and poor functional outcomes. These results give credence to the argument that a high postischemic stroke BP is associated with unfavorable clinical outcomes.

Blood Pressure Management in Acute Ischemic Stroke

As stated previously, multiple observational studies exist demonstrating that BP declines in the first several days following ischemic stroke without pharmacologic intervention.[7,25,26] However, controversy still remains regarding whether it is optimal to actively intervene to pharmacologically lower or increase BP following AIS or to leave it untreated until it exceeds defined upper or lower thresholds.[16]

Few studies have examined the impact of BP reduction in patients with AIS. In 2008, an updated Cochrane review was published to assess the effect of actively intervening to alter BP in patients with AIS on functional outcomes or death. Twelve small randomized studies, including a total of 1153 patients with stroke, were analyzed in the review; the investigators concluded that there was insufficient evidence to determine an effect of lowering BP on clinical outcomes.[27] In the time since that publication, 3 large studies have provided further data.

The Controlling Hypertension and Hypotension Immediately Post-Stroke (CHHIPS) trial was a randomized, placebo-controlled, double-blind study that compared labetalol, lisinopril, and placebo for lowering of BP in 179 patients with either cerebral infarction or primary ICH and an SBP greater than 160 mm Hg. BP was reduced by 21 mm Hg in the active treatment group versus 11 mm Hg in the placebo group; however, there was no significant difference in primary outcome of death or dependency at 2 weeks. Although there was no increase in serious adverse events in the treatment arm, the secondary outcome measure of 3-month mortality was reduced from 20.3% to 9.7% (hazard ratio 0.40, 95% confidence interval [CI] 0.2–1.0).[28]

The angiotensin-receptor blocker candesartan for treatment of acute stroke (SCAST) trial examined whether BP lowering treatment with candesartan was beneficial to patients with acute stroke with increased BP. The trial included 2029 patients with stroke (approximately 85% ischemic, 15% hemorrhagic) and randomized them to receive either candesartan or placebo for 7 days. More than 25% of patients enrolled also received concomitant therapy with antihypertensive agents at the physicians' discretion. A minimal but statistically significant BP lowering effect was seen, with the SBP 5 mm Hg lower in the candesartan group at day 7 compared with the placebo group. No significant difference in death, myocardial infarction, or recurrent stroke at 6 months was observed between the two groups; a slightly higher risk of poor function outcome was seen in the candesartan group at 6 months.[29]

Recently, He and colleagues[30] evaluated the impact of moderate BP reduction within 48 hours of onset in patients with AIS on death and major disability at 14 days or hospital discharge in the Chinese Antihypertensive Trial in Acute Ischemic Stroke (CATIS) trial. This trial is the largest to date evaluating BP lowering in patients with AIS, with 2038 patients assigned to receive antihypertensive agents and 2033 patients in the control group. The patients randomized had SBP between 140 and less than 220 mm Hg at the time of randomization. Exclusion criteria included patients who qualified for thrombolysis and patients with heart failure, acute myocardial infarction or unstable angina, atrial fibrillation, aortic dissection, cerebrovascular stenosis, deep coma, or resistant hypertension. The BP goals in the intervention group were to lower SBP by 10% to 25% within the first 24 hours and to achieve a BP of less than 140/90 within 7 days. The patients enrolled had a median National Institutes of Health Stroke Scale (NIHSS) score of 4. The first-line intervention was intravenous angiotensin-converting enzyme inhibitors followed by calcium channel blockers (second-line) and diuretics (third-line). Patients in the control group were not allowed BP treatment except in extreme circumstances. Within 24 hours, the mean SBP was reduced by 21.8 mm Hg (12.7%) in the treatment group and 12.7 mm Hg (7.2%) in the control group (difference −9.1 mm Hg, $P<.001$) At day 7, the mean SBP in the treatment group was 137.3 mm Hg (65.7% achieved goal BP), whereas the control group mean SBP was 146.5 mm Hg (32.2% achieve goal BP). Finally at day 14, the mean SBP was 135.2 mm Hg (72% achieved goal BP) compared with 143.7 mm Hg (39.5% achieved goal BP) in the control group. The mean differences in SBP between the two groups at day 7 and 14 were −9.3 mm Hg and −8.6 mm Hg, respectively ($P<.001$). Even with this significant difference in BP, no difference was seen in death or major disability at 2 weeks or at 3 months. This trial follows the current guideline recommendation that unless patients qualify for thrombolysis or have BP greater than 220/120 mm Hg, the decision to lower BP acutely does not improve outcomes and should be based on individual clinical judgment if patients have other comorbidities.[16] However, larger trials with well-defined criteria are needed to establish the optimal BP threshold.

Debate also exists regarding whether to continue or withhold antihypertensive medications that patients were receiving before admission. The Continue Or Stop post-Stroke Antihypertensives Collaborative Study (COSSACS) assessed the efficacy and safety of continuing or stopping preexisting antihypertensive medications in patients who had a stroke. Patients were randomized to continue (n = 379; 67% ischemic stroke) or stop (n = 384; 58% ischemic stroke) their preexisting antihypertensive drug within 48 hours of symptom onset. The difference in SBP at 2 weeks between the groups was 13 mm Hg (95% CI 10–17 mm Hg). However, no difference was observed in the primary outcome of death or dependency at 2 weeks. Although this study provides initial data suggesting that continuing prior antihypertensive medications is safe, the results of this study should be taken with caution because COSSACS was underpowered because of the early termination of the trial and patients with dysphagia were excluded, making most of the patients included those with a mild stroke (median NIHSS score of 4).[31]

The most recent trial, Efficacy of Nitric Oxide in Stroke (ENOS), tested whether transdermal glyceryl trinitrate (5 mg for 1 week) is safe and effective in lowering BP and improving outcomes following stroke (4000 patients with AIS and ICH). Patients with baseline SBP of 140 to 220 mm Hg were randomized to active treatment glyceryl trinitrate (5 mg for 1 week), continuing premorbid antihypertensive therapy, or stopping their medication. This trial assessed 2 central concepts: the role of glyceryl trinitrate as a nitric oxide donor to lower BP in the acute phase of stroke and the value of continuing or stopping preexisting antihypertensive agents for 1 week after the stroke.[32] The results of the study were presented at the XXII European Stroke Conference in May 2014. They found that there was a neutral effect on modified Rankin score at 90 days with the use of glyceryl trinitrate, but some benefit was reported in patients treated within 6 hours of symptom onset. The median time to symptom onset was 26 hours, and there was no differential effect seen in patients with AIS and ICH. Patients who received glyceryl trinitrate had higher rates of hypotension and headache. When assessing the role of continuing versus stopping a preexisting antihypertensive agent, they found similar results as COSSACS, with no difference in modified Rankin score at 90 days. However, the secondary analysis found an increase in pneumonia (in patients with dysphagia), disability and cognitive impairment in patients who continued their medications. Unlike the COSSACS trial, ENOS did enroll patients with dysphagia, which illustrates important considerations clinically as there seems to be no urgency in restarting treatment within the first week and safe swallowing should be established before restarting any oral medication.[33]

There are limited data describing the most optimal intravenous antihypertensive to use in the acute stroke setting. Liu-DeRyke and colleagues[34,35] evaluated the therapeutic response and tolerability of labetalol and nicardipine following acute stroke in 2 comparative studies. Both studies enrolled patients according to the American Heart Association/American Stroke Association's (AHA/ASA) guidelines for requiring treatment and assessed patients for the first 24 hours in a mixed stroke population. The first study was a retrospective nonrandomized study that assessed MAP reduction and BP variability differences between labetalol and nicardipine. Most of the patients were experiencing ICH, with 19% in the nicardipine group and 25% in the labetalol group experiencing an AIS. Patients who received nicardipine were more likely to achieve their MAP goals within 1 hour than patients who received labetalol. Secondarily, patients treated with nicardipine required fewer dosage adjustments or need for rescue therapy with additional antihypertensive agents than those who received labetalol.

As a follow-up to this study, the same investigators enrolled 54 patients prospectively in a pseudorandomized study where 35% of patients presented with AIS. Patients received either labetalol or nicardipine for the first 24 hours from admission. The investigators found that the nicardipine group achieved a higher rate of goal BP within 60 minutes of drug initiation, had better maintenance of BP, and a greater percentage of time spent within the goal BP range. None of the patients randomized to nicardipine required rescue medication, whereas 72.7% of those randomized to labetalol required an additional agent to achieve BP goals.[35]

Blood Pressure Management in Patients Eligible for Thrombolytic Therapy

Despite unclear data concerning BP management in patients with general AIS, BP lowering is clearly recommended above certain thresholds for patients with AIS who are eligible to receive thrombolytic therapy.

A pilot study evaluating the factors associated with ICH formation following the use of thrombolytic therapy found that an increased risk of ICH was associated with elevated diastolic BP.[36] Therefore, in the National Institute of Neurologic Disorders and Stroke (NINDS) study, a strict BP of less than 185/110 mm Hg was required for enrollment into the study and tight BP control was maintained for 24 hours with a BP goal of less than 180/105 mm Hg.[37]

Although subsequent observational studies evaluating the association of elevated BP and ICH formation have been variable,[38] a study examining associations between protocol violations and outcomes in community-based recombinant tissue plasminogen activator (rt-PA) use found that when the NINDS protocol is strictly followed, hemorrhage rates are similar to those in the NINDS trial.[39] Furthermore, in 2009 Ahmed and colleagues[40] published results from the Safe Implementation of Thrombolysis in Stroke registry evaluating the association of BP and antihypertensive therapy with clinical outcomes after thrombolytic therapy. The registry included 11,080 patients and categorized patients based on their history of hypertension and whether they were treated with antihypertensives following thrombolysis. Increased SBP 2 to 24 hours after thrombolytic therapy was associated with worse outcome (symptomatic hemorrhage, mortality, functional dependence) at 3 months. The best outcomes were observed in patients with SBP values between 141 and 150 mm Hg up to 24 hours after thrombolysis.

There is an ongoing international trial, Enhanced Control of Hypertension and Thrombolysis Study, that compares a low dose versus a normal dose of rt-PA and intensive BP reduction versus standard reduction in patients receiving thrombolysis. This study will attempt to answer the following 4 key questions: (1) Does low-dose (0.6 mg/kg) intravenous rt-PA provide equivalent benefits compared with the standard dose (0.9 mg/kg) rtPA? (2) Does intensive BP lowering (130–140 mm Hg SBP target) improve outcomes compared with the current guideline-recommended level of BP control (180 mm Hg SBP target)? (3) Does low-dose (0.6 mg/kg) intravenous rt-PA reduce the risk of symptomatic ICH? (4) Does the addition of intensive BP lowering to thrombolysis with rt-PA reduce the risk of any ICH?[41]

It is also important to note that thrombolytic therapy may be associated with improvement in SBP following successful recanalization. Mattle and colleagues[9] reported that patients who underwent intra-arterial thrombolysis and had unsuccessful vessel recanalization had higher and sustained elevations in SBP compared with those patients with successful recanalization.

The AHA/ASA's current guidelines for the management of AIS recommend the use of labetalol and nicardipine as the first-line agents, although there are limited data to support this recommendation. Martin-Schild and colleagues[42] also conducted a retrospective observational study of standard versus aggressive BP management in patients with AIS receiving rt-PA. Standard therapy consisted of labetalol, whereas aggressive therapy consisted of labetalol plus nicardipine or nicardipine alone. Standard and aggressive BP-lowering therapies were equally effective in reaching target BP goals in 3 hours; however, patients receiving aggressive BP lowering had a significantly shorter hospital length of stay (4 days vs 7 days; $P = .01$) than those given labetalol alone.

Minimizing Blood Pressure Variability

BP variability has also become an important monitoring parameter while trying to optimize outcomes in patients with AIS. Stead and colleagues[20] evaluated the impact of acute BP variability following the onset of ischemic stroke. The study cohort consisted of 71 patients, and BP measurements were obtained every 5 minutes throughout the patients' stay in the emergency department. The investigators found that a wide fluctuation in BP (median of 44.5 mm Hg vs 25.0 mm Hg) was associated with an increased risk of death at 90 days. The VISTA collaboration reported that increased SBP variability over 24 hours was significantly associated with poor late functional outcomes, whereas diastolic BP variability did not have an impact on outcomes.[23] Kang and colleagues[43] showed that variability of BP, but not the average BP in the subacute stage (within 48 hours of onset) of AIS, is associated with poor 3-month functional outcomes.

Similar results have been seen when evaluating patients who received thrombolytic therapy. In a study consisting of 80 patients with AIS who received thrombolytic therapy, multiple repeated BP measurements were obtained during the 24 hours following admission. The mean SBP variability was 14.7 ± 5.6 mm Hg. BP variability was found to be associated with greater diffusion-weighted imaging lesion grown and worse clinical outcomes.[44] Comparable results were also shown in a registry trial composed of 527 patients with stroke who received intravenous rt-PA. Patients had their BP measured 8 times within the first 25 hours. The investigators found that early SBP variability was positively associated with ICH and death.[45]

It is important to consider when evaluating these data that BP variability may be a result of stroke severity and, thus, lead to poor functional outcomes because a deteriorating clinical course can result in a variable BP profile; however, most studies did control for stroke severity in their analysis. The Blood Pressure Variability in Acute Ischemic Stroke trial is currently enrolling to evaluate a comparison of BP variability indices and ambulatory arterial stiffness index as prognostic indicators in functional outcomes after AIS.[46]

Minimal literature exist assessing the impact of the various antihypertensive agents on BP variability. However, the 2 trials published by Liu-DeRyke and colleagues[34,35] also reported that nicardipine was associated with less BP variability than labetalol. Future studies describing intravenous antihypertensives following AIS should include an assessment of BP variability.

Induced Hypertension

Adding to the complexity of optimal BP management in patients with AIS, a few studies have suggested a benefit in increasing the BP. Olsen and colleagues[47] demonstrated that increasing the systemic BP can restore cerebral blood flow to the brain and increase perfusion to the ischemic penumbra. However, they also stated that the risk of the development of cerebral edema may outweigh the benefit.

Several small pilot studies have further assessed the outcomes associated with elevating the systemic BP with vasopressor agents. Rordorf and colleagues[48] performed a prospective study that elevated BP in patients with AIS treated within 12 hours of onset. The BP was increased using intravenous phenylephrine until a threshold was found where neurologic deficits improved. Responses were observed in 30% to 50% of the patients treated, and improvements in neurologic deficits were seen within minutes of elevating the BP.

A subsequent pilot study prospectively randomized patients to either induced hypertension with intravenous phenylephrine or conventional management. An MAP increase of 23% was seen in patients being treated with induced hypertension, and these patients demonstrated a reduction in neurologic deficits.[49]

Despite these positive results, concerns still exist regarding the potential adverse effects of increased BP after ischemic stroke, particularly the risk of ICH and worsening cerebral edema. Additionally, vasopressor use may result in cardiac arrhythmias and renal insufficiency.[38]

INTRACEREBRAL HEMORRHAGE

Elevated BP is commonly seen in patients presenting with acute ICH; however, there is continued debate on the best treatment approach. Physiologically, both relative hypotension and continued hypertension could be deleterious. If the BP is lowered too rapidly, one may develop cerebral hypoperfusion with the subsequent development of cerebral ischemia and worsening neurologic status. Conversely, if the BP is allowed to be continuously elevated, the course could be complicated by further hemorrhage or worsening cerebral edema also leading to neurologic decline. The key clinical questions that are reviewed based on the currently available evidence include the following: (1) Does aggressive BP reduction reduce the risk of hematoma expansion? (2) Does BP reduction lead to cerebral hypoperfusion and ischemia? (3) What is the optimal BP goal in patients with ICH and hypertension?

Abnormal Blood Pressure in Intracerebral Hemorrhage

An acute elevation in BP is commonly seen in the setting of ICH, with approximately 70% of patients having an SBP greater than 140 mm Hg within 1 hour of presentation.[5] A history of hypertension has been shown to be associated with an elevated BP on admission.[2,50] In fact, a large population-based study performed in the United Kingdom demonstrated that the SBP is increased substantially in comparison with the premorbid BP in patients with ICH.[10] Furthermore, several studies have demonstrated that patients with elevated BP on admission or within the first 24 hours have an increased risk of death and severe disability after ICH.[51–53] Hypotension on admission has also been found to be associated with worse outcomes, with 52% of those admitted with an SBP less than 100 mm Hg having an early neurologic decline.[54] Cardiovascular disease was the most common cause of death in these cases, as these patients commonly had preexisting heart failure and coronary artery disease.[19]

Hematoma Expansion

Patients with ICH are at risk for hematoma expansion and an associated neurologic decline. In observational studies, up to 38% of patients have a substantial increase in the volume of the hematoma within the first 24 hours, and neurologic decline is more common in this group of patients.[55] Although several factors have been associated with hematoma expansion, elevated BP seems to have the strongest association across several studies.[56–59] Additionally, analysis of the intensive blood pressure reduction in acute cerebral hemorrhage Trial (INTERACT) trial data demonstrated a reduction of hematoma enlargement in one-third of participants when the lowest target BP was achieved within the first 24 hours[60] and overall BP reduction was shown to attenuate hematoma enlargement at 72 hours.[61] However, in the larger INTERACT2 study, no difference in hematoma expansion was noted between the groups after adjustment for prognostic variables.[62]

Perihematomal Cerebral Perfusion and Ischemia

Severely elevated BP in the setting of ICH is likely multifactorial; however, concerns about rapid reduction in BP leading to neurologic decline has been a clinical concern. Those with long-standing hypertension may have a shift in the range for cerebral autoregulation, and acutely reducing the BP to less than that range may lead to autoregulatory failure and cerebral ischemia.[63,64] Furthermore, early studies raised the concern that the brain immediately surrounding the hematoma may be at risk for ischemia from reduced blood flow when the BP is reduced acutely.[65–67] However, subsequent studies using various imaging modalities have not supported these findings. Powers and colleagues[68] demonstrated that global and periclot cerebral blood flow does not change with acute reduction in BP by 17 mm Hg in patients with small-to moderate-sized hematoma volumes. Additionally, studies using computed tomography (CT) perfusion indicate that the perihematomal region has adequate perfusion and is without a penumbra.[69–72] The study performed by Butcher and colleagues,[70] the Intracerebral Hemorrhage Acutely Decreasing Arterial Pressure Trial, was a randomized trial that enrolled 75 patients with ICH and SBP greater than 150 mm Hg to protocol-guided antihypertensive therapy with a goal of less than 150 mm Hg versus less than 180 mm Hg. The primary outcome was the relative change in perihematomal cerebral blood flow as measured using CT perfusion. Although BP was lower with 2 hours after randomization in the less than 150 mm Hg target group, there was no significant difference in the relative change in perihematomal cerebral blood flow in this group when compared with the less than 180 mm Hg target group. Furthermore, there was no relationship between the amount of reduction in BP and the perihematomal relative cerebral blood flow for those subjects in either of the groups. These data further indicate that rapid lowering of the BP in patients with ICH and elevated BP will not precipitate perihematomal cerebral ischemia. Given the results of these studies, several clinical trials have been completed or are ongoing evaluating the safety and efficacy of BP reduction in the setting of ICH.

Blood Pressure Control and Intracerebral Hemorrhage

Because of the association between stroke and elevated BP on admission as well as during hospitalization, several studies have been performed to determine if BP control in the acute setting would improve outcomes in this population. Several of these clinical trials have included patients with AIS or ICH, whereas others have focused strictly on patients with ICH. Three of the largest trials completed that enrolled patients with both types of stroke include CHHIPS, COSSACS, and SCAST.[28,29,31]

The trials in this group, CHHIPS, COSSACS, and SCAST, were previously described. However, these studies have limited insight into the ICH population. Only 43 patients with ICH were enrolled in CHHIPS, and the placebo arm only included 7 patients in the ICH subgroup.

Therefore, the interpretation of these results in this population is very limited.[28] COSSACS included only 38 patients with ICH, and it too cannot provide adequate data as to the safety and efficacy of BP reduction after ICH.[31] There were 274 patients with ICH randomized in SCAST; subgroup analyses of this group did not identify any significant effect for the prescribed outcomes.[29]

As described earlier, preliminary results from the recently completed ENOS trial have been presented. Although the complete results have yet to be published, this trial included 629 participants with ICH; hence, the results for this subgroup are highly anticipated.[32]

Because of the association of BP elevation with ICH and the potential risk of neurologic decline caused by hematoma expansion, several clinical trials have been performed over the past decade with the goal of determining whether BP reduction is safe and efficacious. INTERACT was a randomized study that enrolled 404 patients to either intensive BP reduction with a goal SBP of 140 mm Hg versus standard guideline-based management with a goal SBP of 180 mm Hg. The primary end point was change in hematoma volume at 24 hours, and the secondary outcomes included safety and clinical outcomes at 90 days. The BP was significantly lower in the intensive group from 1 hour after enrollment until 24 hours, whereas mean proportional hematoma growth was significantly less at 13.7% versus 36.3% for the guideline group. There were no reported differences between groups in the 90-day clinical and safety outcomes. Although a reduction in hematoma volume was noted in this trial, the absolute difference was only 1.7 mL, which may not be clinically meaningful.[73]

The antihypertensive treatment of acute cerebral hemorrhage (ATACH) trial was a relatively small phase I dose-escalation study aimed at determining the feasibility and safety of reducing BP in patients with ICH and SBP of greater than 170 mm Hg. Although the INTERACT study allowed for local sites to decide on which antihypertensive agents to use, the ATACH study has a prescribed algorithm for BP reduction using intravenous nicardipine. SBP reduction was tiered, with the first 18 patients having a target of 170 to 200 mm Hg, the next 20 patients having a target of 140 to 170 mm Hg, and the last having a target of 110 to 140 mm Hg. Although aggressive BP reduction was feasible, 9 of the 22 patients in the most aggressive reduction arm were treatment failures suggesting that their protocol was not optimal for such aggressive BP reduction. Additionally, although there were a larger proportion of patients with neurologic decline or serious adverse events in the most aggressive tier, the safety-stopping rule was not met for any of the groups. The study was not powered to determine differences in clinical outcome, which were no different between study arms.[74] The INTERACT and ATACH trials were preliminary studies to determine the feasibility of the selected BP targets as well as safety. Neither study was powered to determine if BP reduction was efficacious for clinical outcomes. Based on the analysis of each study, larger randomized trials with similar study designs were undertaken, INTERACT2 and ATACH II.

INTERACT2 was a prospective, randomized, open-treatment, blinded end-point trial aimed at determining if aggressive BP reduction in patients with ICH and BP elevation would improve clinical outcomes. Participants were enrolled within 6 hours of onset and were randomly assigned to receive either intensive BP reduction with a goal SBP of less than 140 mm Hg or guideline-recommended treatment with a goal SBP of less than 180 mm Hg. The primary outcome was death or major disability (score of 3–6 on the modified Rankin scale), and a prespecified ordinal analysis of the modified Rankin scale was also performed as the main secondary outcome. The ordinal analysis was added as a secondary outcome after completion of enrollment but before data analysis. This analysis allows for the statistical analysis to determine if there is a significant shift in the distribution of clinical outcomes an ordinal scale such as the modified Rankin scale. Although the mean SBP did differ between the two groups from 15 minutes to 7 days, 150 mm Hg in the intensive-treatment group versus 164 mm Hg in the guideline-treatment group, only 33.4% of patients achieved the target BP in the intensive-treatment group. There was no difference in the primary outcome between the two treatment groups, whereas the ordinal analysis showed a significantly lower modified Rankin scale score with an odds ratio of 0.87 for greater disability (P = .04) in the aggressive-treatment arm. Furthermore, there was no difference in mortality or serious adverse events between the two arms of the study.[62]

ATACH II is an ongoing prospective randomized trial with a planned enrollment of 1280 subjects with ICH and an SBP greater than 180 mm Hg. Participants will be randomized to either a target SBP of less than 180 mm Hg or less than 140 mm Hg using a prespecified antihypertensive algorithm using continuous infusion of intravenous nicardipine. Treatment will begin within 3 hours of onset and continued for 24 hours. The primary outcome is death or disability (modified Rankin score 4–6) at 3 months with secondary outcomes including quality of life measures at 3 months, hematoma expansion at 24 hours, as well as treatment-related serious adverse events within the first 72 hours. Although this study is not projected to be complete until July 2016, the findings should further assist clinicians in determining the safest and most efficacious treatment of this population.[75]

Continued Controversies

Although much effort and funding has been put into the study of ICH, there continue to be areas of controversy surrounding the optimal management of the hypertensive response seen in patients with ICH. Two of the main areas of controversy have included the risk of perihematomal ischemia with BP reduction as well as the optimal BP targets that would improve clinical outcomes.

The concern for perihematomal ischemia has been well addressed in numerous studies.[67–71,76] Although there may be individual cases of perihematomal reduction in cerebral blood flow and ischemia identified, we should feel confident that the reduction of BP does not lead to significant perihematomal ischemia when evaluated in prospective studies. Furthermore, the INTERACT, ATACH, and INTERACT2 studies did not demonstrate a significant neurologic decline with aggressive BP reduction when compared with guideline-based treatment.[62,73,74] Clinicians may be faced with the case of a perfusion-dependent clinical examination that is assumed to be caused by perihematomal ischemia; in this rare case, clinical judgment would be necessary in light of the data that exist.

Even though we now have several clinical trials aimed at answering the question of what BP target is safe and efficacious for patients with ICH and hypertension, the answer is unfortunately still not clear. Although none of the trials to date have found BP reduction to improve clinical outcomes, these trials did not demonstrate any harm in aggressive BP reduction. Without further data, aggressive BP reduction is not supported by the current literature. Aggressive BP reduction may lead to an overall increased cost of providing care to this patient population through an increase in intensive-care-unit admissions and a longer length of hospital stay.

INTERACT2 failed to show a benefit for aggressive BP reduction in improving clinical outcome; however, post hoc analysis has raised the issue of whether BP variability may have affected the outcome measurement in the aggressive BP reduction arm. When BP standard deviation was evaluated during the hyperacute (first 24 hours) and acute (days 2–7) phase, a significant linear association was found with the primary outcome. Furthermore, the strongest predictor for outcomes during the acute phase of BP control was the standard deviation of the SBP.[77] Although the outcome in INTERACT2 may have been affected by significant fluctuations in BP, the ongoing ATACH II study may help address this issue because of its use of continuous infusion nicardipine for BP control. However, the infusion is only for the initial 24 hours;

therefore, if BP variability affects outcome after this hyperacute period, then this question may remained unanswered.[75]

SUMMARY

Questions remain regarding the optimal BP management in the hyperacute period following acute stroke. Complexities yet to be resolved include whether acute elevations in BP are physiologic and protective or are a result of the stress reaction that is harmful to the brain and whether lowering BP is beneficial. Adequately powered randomized trials are needed to help resolve these remaining conundrums.

Although the decision to initiate acute antihypertensive therapy has not been clearly delineated, the current evidence suggests that, in most patients with AIS who do not qualify for thrombolysis, antihypertensives can be safely withheld early except when the BP exceeds 220/120 mm Hg or in the presence of another acute, severe, and compelling indication, such as aortic dissection or myocardial infarction (T3, 3-0). The CATIS subgroup analysis of the time to randomization suggests that patients with mild AIS had better 6-month outcomes when BP lowering was withheld the first 12 hours and beyond 24 hours.[30] This finding suggests that reinitiation of antihypertensives in the 12- to 36-hour period following stroke may be beneficial (T2, 2-1). However, considerations should be made regarding the route of administration in dysphagic patients with avoidance of oral agents until swallowing can be established based on the initial results from the ENOS trial (T2, 3-X).

For patients who qualify for thrombolysis, the current recommendations are that BP that is elevated more than 185/110 mm Hg should be carefully lowered before initiation of thrombolysis (T1, 1-1). For the first 24 hours after treatment, BP should be maintained at less than 180/105 mm Hg (T1, 1-1). When treatment is initiated, an agent should be selected that has rapid onset of action and that is titratable in order to avoid BP variability because BP variability seems to be linked to poor functional outcomes and an increased risk of hemorrhagic transformation of the infarct (T2, 2-1). The impact of the agent on comorbidities, heart rate, and intracranial pressure should also be considered. No large direct comparison trial has evaluated which of these antihypertensive agents is superior in clinical outcomes.

As in AIS, BP elevation is common in patients presenting with spontaneous ICH. Although early studies suggested an increased risk of perihematomal hypoperfusion and ischemia with BP reduction, multiple prospective follow-up studies have demonstrated that BP reduction does not lead to perihematomal hypoperfusion and ischemia (T3, 3-1).

Conversely, previous data have demonstrated that elevated BP is associated with hematoma expansion in patients with ICH and that aggressive BP reduction is not only safe but also leads to a reduction in hematoma expansion.[73] However, the INTERACT2 trial did not demonstrate a reduction in hematoma expansion as a secondary end point; therefore, based on the best available data, aggressive BP reduction does not reduce the risk of hematoma expansion versus standard management using the current guidelines (T1, 1-0).[78]

BP control in the setting of ICH has been evaluated in several randomized prospective studies with clinically meaningful end points. Based on the current literature, although it seems safe, aggressive BP reduction less than the AHA/ASA's current guideline target of SBP less than 180 to 200 mm Hg is not supported (T1, 1-0).

REFERENCES

1. Wallace JD, Levy LL. Blood pressure after stroke. JAMA 1981;246(19):2177–80.

2. Britton M, Carlsson A, de Faire U. Blood pressure course in patients with acute stroke and matched controls. Stroke 1986;17(5):861–4.
3. CAST (Chinese Acute Stroke Trial) Collaborative Group. CAST: randomised placebo-controlled trial of early aspirin use in 20,000 patients with acute ischaemic stroke. Lancet 1997;349(9066):1641–9.
4. International Stroke Trial Collaborative Group. The International Stroke Trial (IST): a randomised trial of aspirin, subcutaneous heparin, both, or neither among 19435 patients with acute ischaemic stroke. Lancet 1997;349(9065):1569–81.
5. Qureshi AI, Ezzeddine MA, Nasar A, et al. Prevalence of elevated blood pressure in 563,704 adult patients with stroke presenting to the ED in the United States. Am J Emerg Med 2007;25(1):32–8.
6. Harper G, Castleden CM, Potter JF. Factors affecting changes in blood pressure after acute stroke. Stroke 1994;25(9):1726–9.
7. Broderick J, Brott T, Barsan W, et al. Blood pressure during the first minutes of focal cerebral ischemia. Ann Emerg Med 1993;22(9):1438–43.
8. Chamorro A, Vila N, Ascaso C, et al. Blood pressure and functional recovery in acute ischemic stroke. Stroke 1998;29(9):1850–3.
9. Mattle HP, Kappeler L, Arnold M, et al. Blood pressure and vessel recanalization in the first hours after ischemic stroke. Stroke 2005;36(2):264–8.
10. Fischer U, Cooney MT, Bull LM, et al. Acute post-stroke blood pressure relative to premorbid levels in intracerebral haemorrhage versus major ischaemic stroke: a population-based study. Lancet Neurol 2014;13(4):374–84.
11. Strandgaard S, Paulson OB. Cerebral autoregulation. Stroke 1984;15(3):413–6.
12. Paulson OB, Strandgaard S, Edvinsson L. Cerebral autoregulation. Cerebrovasc Brain Metab Rev 1990;2(2):161–92.
13. Lang EW, Lagopoulos J, Griffith J, et al. Cerebral vasomotor reactivity testing in head injury: the link between pressure and flow. J Neurol Neurosurg Psychiatr 2003;74(8):1053–9.
14. Jordan JD, Powers WJ. Cerebral autoregulation and acute ischemic stroke. Am J Hypertens 2012;25(9):946–50.
15. Varon J, Marik PE. The diagnosis and management of hypertensive crises. Chest 2000;118(1):214–27.
16. Jauch EC, Saver JL, Adams HP, et al. American Heart Association Stroke Council, Council on Cardiovascular Nursing, Council on Peripheral Vascular Disease, Council on Clinical Cardiology. Guidelines for the early management of patients with acute ischemic stroke: a guideline for healthcare professionals from the American Heart Association/American Stroke Association. Stroke 2013;44(3): 870–947.
17. Hornig CR, Dorndorf W, Agnoli AL. Hemorrhagic cerebral infarction—a prospective study. Stroke 1986;17(2):179–85.
18. Leonardi-Bee J, Bath PM, Phillips SJ, et al, IST Collaborative Group. Blood pressure and clinical outcomes in the International Stroke Trial. Stroke 2002;33(5): 1315–20.
19. Vemmos KN, Spengos K, Tsivgoulis G, et al. Factors influencing acute blood pressure values in stroke subtypes. J Hum Hypertens 2004;18(4):253–9.
20. Stead LG, Gilmore RM, Vedula KC, et al. Impact of acute blood pressure variability on ischemic stroke outcome. Neurology 2006;66(12):1878–81.
21. Ahmed N, Wahlgren G. High initial blood pressure after acute stroke is associated with poor functional outcome. J Intern Med 2001;249(5):467–73.
22. Jensen MB, Yoo B, Clarke WR, et al. Blood pressure as an independent prognostic factor in acute ischemic stroke. Can J Neurol Sci 2006;33(1):34–8.

23. Sare GM, Ali M, Shuaib A, et al, for the VISTA Collaboration. Relationship between hyperacute blood pressure and outcome after ischemic stroke: data from the VISTA collaboration. Stroke 2009;40(6):2098–103.
24. Ishitsuka K, Kamouchi M, Hata J, et al, FSR Investigators. High blood pressure after acute ischemic stroke is associated with poor clinical outcomes: Fukuoka Stroke Registry. Hypertension 2014;63(1):54–60.
25. Schrader J, Lüders S, Kulschewski A, et al, Acute Candesartan Cilexetil Therapy in Stroke Survivors Study Group. The ACCESS Study: evaluation of Acute Candesartan Cilexetil Therapy in Stroke Survivors. Stroke 2003;34(7):1699–703.
26. Aslanyan S, Fazekas F, Weir CJ, et al, GAIN International Steering Committee and Investigators. Effect of blood pressure during the acute period of ischemic stroke on stroke outcome: a tertiary analysis of the GAIN International Trial. Stroke 2003; 34(10):2420–5.
27. Geeganage C, Bath PM. Interventions for deliberately altering blood pressure in acute stroke. Cochrane Database Syst Rev 2008;(4):CD000039.
28. Potter JF, Robinson TG, Ford GA, et al. Controlling hypertension and hypotension immediately post-stroke (CHHIPS): a randomised, placebo-controlled, double-blind pilot trial. Lancet Neurol 2009;8(1):48–56.
29. Sandset EC, Bath PM, Boysen G, et al, SCAST Study Group. The angiotensin-receptor blocker candesartan for treatment of acute stroke (SCAST): a randomised, placebo-controlled, double-blind trial. Lancet 2011;377(9767):741–50.
30. He J, Zhang Y, Xu T, et al. Effects of immediate blood pressure reduction on death and major disability in patients with acute ischemic stroke. JAMA 2014;311(5): 479–89.
31. Robinson TG, Potter JF, Ford GA, et al, COSSACS Investigators. Effects of anti-hypertensive treatment after acute stroke in the Continue or Stop post-Stroke Antihypertensives Collaborative Study (COSSACS): a prospective, randomised, open, blinded-endpoint trial. Lancet Neurol 2010;9(8):767–75.
32. ENOS Investigators. Baseline characteristics of the 4011 patients recruited into the "Efficacy of Nitric Oxide in Stroke" (ENOS) trial. Int J Stroke 2014;9(6):711–20.
33. Hughes S. ENOS: no rush to continue oral BP meds in acute stroke. Medscape 2014.
34. Liu-DeRyke X, Janisse J, Coplin WM, et al. A Comparison of nicardipine and labetalol for acute hypertension management following stroke. Neurocrit Care 2008;9(2):167–76.
35. Liu-DeRyke X, Levy PD, Parker D, et al. A prospective evaluation of labetalol versus nicardipine for blood pressure management in patients with acute stroke. Neurocrit Care 2013;19(1):41–7.
36. Levy DE, Brott TG, Haley EC, et al. Factors related to intracranial hematoma formation in patients receiving tissue-type plasminogen activator for acute ischemic stroke. Stroke 1994;25(2):291–7.
37. Tissue plasminogen activator for acute ischemic stroke. The National Institute of Neurological Disorders and Stroke rt-PA Stroke Study Group. N Engl J Med 1995; 333(24):1581–7.
38. Wityk RJ, Lewin JJ. Blood pressure management during acute ischaemic stroke. Expert Opin Pharmacother 2006;7(3):247–58.
39. Lopez-Yunez AM, Bruno A, Williams LS, et al. Protocol violations in community-based rTPA stroke treatment are associated with symptomatic intracerebral hemorrhage. Stroke 2001;32(1):12–6.
40. Ahmed N, Wahlgren N, Brainin M, et al. SITS Investigators. Relationship of blood pressure, antihypertensive therapy, and outcome in ischemic stroke treated with

intravenous thrombolysis: retrospective analysis from Safe Implementation of Thrombolysis in Stroke-International Stroke Thrombolysis Register (SITS-ISTR). Stroke 2009;40(7):2442–9.

41. Enhanced Control of Hypertension and Thrombolysis Stroke Study (ENCHANTED). http://clinicaltrials.gov/show/NCT01422616. Accessed December 01, 2014.

42. Martin-Schild S, Hallevi H, Albright KC, et al. Aggressive blood pressure-lowering treatment before intravenous tissue plasminogen activator therapy in acute ischemic stroke. Arch Neurol 2008;65(9):1174–8.

43. Kang J, Ko Y, Park JH, et al. Effect of blood pressure on 3-month functional outcome in the subacute stage of ischemic stroke. Neurology 2012;79(20): 2018–24.

44. Delgado-Mederos R, Ribo M, Rovira A, et al. Prognostic significance of blood pressure variability after thrombolysis in acute stroke. Neurology 2008;71(8):552–8.

45. Endo K, Kario K, Koga M, et al. Impact of early blood pressure variability on stroke outcomes after thrombolysis: the SAMURAI rt-PA Registry. Stroke 2013; 44(3):816–8.

46. Blood pressure variability in acute ischemic stroke (PREVISE). http://clinicaltrials. gov/show/NCT01915862. Accessed December 01, 2014.

47. Olsen TS, Larsen B, Herning M, et al. Blood flow and vascular reactivity in collaterally perfused brain tissue. Evidence of an ischemic penumbra in patients with acute stroke. Stroke 1983;14(3):332–41.

48. Rordorf G, Koroshetz WJ, Ezzeddine MA, et al. A pilot study of drug-induced hypertension for treatment of acute stroke. Neurology 2001;56(9):1210–3.

49. Hillis AE, Ulatowski JA, Barker PB, et al. A pilot randomized trial of induced blood pressure elevation: effects on function and focal perfusion in acute and subacute stroke. Cerebrovasc Dis 2003;16(3):236–46.

50. Carlberg B, Asplund K, Hägg E. Factors influencing admission blood pressure levels in patients with acute stroke. Stroke 1991;22(4):527–30.

51. Fogelholm R, Avikainen S, Murros K. Prognostic value and determinants of first-day mean arterial pressure in spontaneous supratentorial intracerebral hemorrhage. Stroke 1997;28(7):1396–400.

52. Carlberg B, Asplund K, Hägg E. The prognostic value of admission blood pressure in patients with acute stroke. Stroke 1993;24(9):1372–5.

53. Vemmos KN, Tsivgoulis G, Spengos K, et al. U-shaped relationship between mortality and admission blood pressure in patients with acute stroke. J Intern Med 2004;255(2):257–65.

54. Ohwaki K, Yano E, Nagashima H, et al. Blood pressure management in acute intracerebral haemorrhage: low blood pressure and early neurological deterioration. Br J Neurosurg 2010;24(4):410–4.

55. Brott T, Broderick J, Kothari R, et al. Early hemorrhage growth in patients with intracerebral hemorrhage. Stroke 1997;28(1):1–5.

56. Ohwaki K, Yano E, Nagashima H, et al. Blood pressure management in acute intracerebral hemorrhage: relationship between elevated blood pressure and hematoma enlargement. Stroke 2004;35(6):1364–7.

57. Broderick JP, Diringer MN, Hill MD, et al, Recombinant Activated Factor VII Intracerebral Hemorrhage Trial Investigators. Determinants of intracerebral hemorrhage growth: an exploratory analysis. Stroke 2007;38(3):1072–5.

58. Rodriguez-Luna D, Piñeiro S, Rubiera M, et al. Impact of blood pressure changes and course on hematoma growth in acute intracerebral hemorrhage. Eur J Neurol 2013;20(9):1277–83.

59. Vemmos KN, Tsivgoulis G, Spengos K, et al. Association between 24-h blood pressure monitoring variables and brain oedema in patients with hyperacute stroke. J Hypertens 2003;21(11):2167–73.
60. Arima H, Anderson CS, Wang JG, et al, Intensive Blood Pressure Reduction in Acute Cerebral Haemorrhage Trial Investigators. Lower treatment blood pressure is associated with greatest reduction in hematoma growth after acute intracerebral hemorrhage. Hypertension 2010;56(5):852–8.
61. Anderson CS, Huang Y, Arima H, et al, INTERACT Investigators. Effects of early intensive blood pressure-lowering treatment on the growth of hematoma and perihematomal edema in acute intracerebral hemorrhage: the Intensive Blood Pressure Reduction in Acute Cerebral Haemorrhage Trial (INTERACT). Stroke 2010; 41(2):307–12.
62. Anderson CS, Heeley E, Huang Y, et al, INTERACT2 Investigators. Rapid blood-pressure lowering in patients with acute intracerebral hemorrhage. N Engl J Med 2013;368(25):2355–65.
63. Strandgaard S. Autoregulation of cerebral blood flow in hypertensive patients. The modifying influence of prolonged antihypertensive treatment on the tolerance to acute, drug-induced hypotension. Circulation 1976;53(4):720–7.
64. Strandgaard S, Olesen J, Skinhoj E, et al. Autoregulation of brain circulation in severe arterial hypertension. Br Med J 1973;1(5852):507–10.
65. Sills C, Villar-Cordova C, Pasteur W, et al. Demonstration of hypoperfusion surrounding intracerebral hematoma in humans. J Stroke Cerebrovasc Dis 1996; 6(1):17–24.
66. Mayer SA, Lignelli A, Fink ME, et al. Perilesional blood flow and edema formation in acute intracerebral hemorrhage: a SPECT study. Stroke 1998;29(9):1791–8.
67. Rosand J, Eskey C, Chang Y, et al. Dynamic single-section CT demonstrates reduced cerebral blood flow in acute intracerebral hemorrhage. Cerebrovasc Dis 2002;14(3–4):214–20.
68. Powers WJ, Zazulia AR, Videen TO, et al. Autoregulation of cerebral blood flow surrounding acute (6 to 22 hours) intracerebral hemorrhage. Neurology 2001; 57(1):18–24.
69. Gould B, McCourt R, Gioia LC, et al, ICH ADAPT Investigators. Acute blood pressure reduction in patients with intracerebral hemorrhage does not result in border zone region hypoperfusion. Stroke 2014;45(10):2894–9.
70. Butcher KS, Jeerakathil T, Hill M, et al, ICH ADAPT Investigators. The intracerebral hemorrhage acutely decreasing arterial pressure trial. Stroke 2013;44(3): 620–6.
71. Herweh C, Jüttler E, Schellinger PD, et al. Evidence against a perihemorrhagic penumbra provided by perfusion computed tomography. Stroke 2007;38(11): 2941–7.
72. Herweh C, Jüttler E, Schellinger PD, et al. Perfusion CT in hyperacute cerebral hemorrhage within 3 hours after symptom onset: is there an early perihemorrhagic penumbra? J Neuroimaging 2010;20(4):350–3.
73. Anderson CS, Huang Y, Wang JG, et al. Intensive blood pressure reduction in acute cerebral haemorrhage trial (INTERACT): a randomised pilot trial. Lancet Neurol 2008;7(5):391–9.
74. Antihypertensive Treatment of Acute Cerebral Hemorrhage ATACH investigators. Antihypertensive treatment of acute cerebral hemorrhage. Crit Care Med 2010; 38(2):637–48.
75. Qureshi AI, Palesch YY. Antihypertensive treatment of acute cerebral hemorrhage (ATACH) II: design, methods, and rationale. Neurocrit Care 2011;15(3):559–76.

76. Olivot JM, Mlynash M, Kleinman JT, et al, DASH investigators. MRI profile of the perihematomal region in acute intracerebral hemorrhage. Stroke 2010;41(11): 2681–3.

77. Manning L, Hirakawa Y, Arima H, et al, INTERACT2 Investigators. Blood pressure variability and outcome after acute intracerebral haemorrhage: a post-hoc analysis of INTERACT2, a randomised controlled trial. Lancet Neurol 2014;13(4): 364–73.

78. Morgenstern LB, Hemphill JC, Anderson C, et al. American Heart Association Stroke Council and Council on Cardiovascular Nursing. Guidelines for the management of spontaneous intracerebral hemorrhage: a guideline for healthcare professionals from the American Heart Association/American Stroke Association. Stroke 2010;41(9):2108–29.

Expansion of Intravenous Tissue Plasminogen Activator Eligibility Beyond National Institute of Neurological Disorders and Stroke and European Cooperative Acute Stroke Study III Criteria

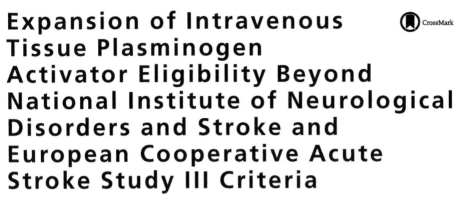 CrossMark

Adrian Marchidann, MD[a,c,*], Clotilde Balucani, MD, PhD[a],
Steven R. Levine, MD[b,c]

KEYWORDS

- Stroke • Treatment • Thrombolysis • tPA • Alteplase • Guidelines • Off-label
- Contraindications

KEY POINTS

- Overall, off-label use of tissue plasminogen activator (tPA) appears to be safe and beneficial for many subgroups of patients with acute ischemic stroke.
- Several former absolute contraindications for tPA have become relative: age older than 80 years, pregnancy, minor or rapidly improving stroke, large stroke, seizures, recent surgery, recent stroke, recent myocardial infarction, and gastrointestinal or urinary hemorrhage.
- Little is known about the safety and efficacy of tPA in patients with uncontrolled hypertension, previous intracerebral hemorrhage, and coagulopathy.
- Further randomized studies could help confirm the safety and efficacy of thrombolysis in patients with absolute and relative contraindications.

Disclosures: Dr A. Marchidann is the local principal investigator for the NINDS-funded POINT (5U01NS062835) trial and contributes updates for MEDLINK. Dr C. Balucani is supported by an Award from the American Heart Association Founders Affiliate and the American Brain Foundation. Dr S.R. Levine is funded by NIH and PCORI, serves on the Scientific Advisory Committee/Steering Committee of PRISMS, a Genentech-funded randomized clinical trial. He also serves as an associate editor for MEDLINK. He has also participated in medical-legal proceedings.
[a] Department of Neurology, SUNY Downstate Medical Center & Stroke Center, 450 Clarkson Avenue, Brooklyn, NY 11203, USA; [b] Department of Neurology, SUNY Downstate Medical Center & Stroke Center, 450 Clarkson Avenue, MSC 1213, Brooklyn, NY 11203, USA; [c] Department of Neurology, The Kings County Hospital Center, 451 Clarkson Avenue, Brooklyn, NY 11203, USA
* Corresponding author. Department of Neurology, SUNY Downstate Medical Center & Stroke Center, 450 Clarkson Avenue, Brooklyn, NY 11203.
E-mail address: adrian.marchidann@downstate.edu

Neurol Clin 33 (2015) 381–400
http://dx.doi.org/10.1016/j.ncl.2015.01.004   **neurologic.theclinics.com**
0733-8619/15/$ – see front matter © 2015 Elsevier Inc. All rights reserved.

THE PROBLEM

Since the publication of the National Institute of Neurological Disorders and Stroke (NINDS) trial results,[1] intravenous (IV) tissue plasminogen activator (tPA) has become the standard treatment of acute ischemic stroke. However, due to many contraindications, only a minority of patients are eligible for and may potentially benefit from it. This article reviews the available data and seeks to expand our knowledge on the potential benefits as well as limitations of IV tPA outside of the guidelines.

REVIEW OF THE AVAILABLE DATA

Stroke is one of the most important causes of morbidity and mortality worldwide. IV administration of tPA within 3 hours of symptom onset is currently the only Food and Drug Administration (FDA)-approved drug treatment of acute ischemic stroke in the United States. In 2009, only 3.4% to 5.2% of patients with acute stroke received IV tPA in the United States.[2] Adherence to the explicit inclusion and exclusion criteria for clinical practice has been the most common protocol for using IV tPA in clinical practice.

With almost 20 years of thrombolysis experience in acute ischemic stroke, clinicians have become more comfortable with treating and weighing individual patient risk-benefit. There has been a growing practice of treating patients outside of published guidelines, specifically with one or more exclusion criteria in both the 0 to 3.0-hour and 3.0 to 4.5-hour treatment window[3] or other medical conditions that may be associated with complications.[4]

In an observational study from a busy emergency department (ED), most patients were ineligible because of delay in treatment, resolution of symptoms, intracerebral hemorrhage (ICH), and minor symptoms.[5] In another study, 73% of patients were excluded because of late presentation. Other reasons were mild stroke, clinical improvement, perceived protocol exclusions, ED referral delay, and significant comorbidities.[6] Chart analysis of patients who had not received thrombolysis despite no documented contraindication (48% of eligible patients) revealed that old age and late presentation were associated with nontreatment.[7]

The European Cooperative Acute Stroke Study (ECASS)[8] and ECASS II,[9] as well as the Alteplase Thrombolysis for Acute Noninterventional Therapy in Ischemic Stroke (ATLANTIS) trials failed to demonstrate significant benefit of tPA given between 0 to 6 hours and 3 to 5 hours, respectively,[10] but they were clearly underpowered for the effect size subsequently seen. A pooled analysis of 6 trials enrolling 2775 patients within the 6-hour window showed benefit of IV tPA up to 4.5 hours, not only in increased rate of excellent outcome, but also in improving outcome along the entire range of poststroke disability. Beyond 4.5 hours, there was increased rate of mortality with no significant clinical benefit.[11]

Perfusion-diffusion weighted (PWI-DWI) MRI mismatch was used to test the benefit of tPA within the 3-hour to 6-hour window. Reperfusion measured at 3 to 5 days was more common with tPA than with placebo in patients with mismatch and was associated with less infarct growth and better neurologic and functional outcome than was lack of reperfusion.[12]

The ECASS III trial confirmed the benefit of tPA administration 3.0 to 4.5 hours from onset of symptoms.[13] A post hoc sampling of data from the Safe Implementation of Thrombolysis in Stroke–International Stroke Treatment Registry (SITS-ISTR) showed no difference between the patients treated within 3 hours and those treated between 3.0 and 4.5 hours with respect to mortality, symptomatic intracerebral hemorrhage (SICH), or good outcome at 90 days.[14] Although the third International Stroke Trial

(IST-3) did not show improved survival and disability in patients who received tPA within 6 hours, secondary ordinal analysis demonstrated that these patients survived with less disability at the 6-month follow-up visit. The benefit did not seem to diminish in elderly patients. Data from the IST-3 trial was incorporated into a systematic review of 12 randomized trials, totalling 7012 patients treated within 6 hours, and was consistent with the results of the previous trials.[15] At 18 months, mortality between the tPA and placebo arms was similar, but the reduction in mortality was greater in patients randomized within 3 hours.[16] Because subgroup analysis showed no benefit within the 4.5-hour to 6.0-hour window, a result supported by a pooled analysis of several major studies, tPA administration beyond 4.5 hours cannot be recommended.[17] However, the yield of the extended therapeutic window is small. A population-based study revealed that only 3.4% of patients arrived in the extended time window and only 0.5% of these were eligible for thrombolysis according to standard criteria.[18]

The effectiveness of thrombolytic therapy clearly diminishes with time. In a pooled analysis of several clinical trials, the adjusted odds of good outcome at 3 months in favor of tPA decreased from 2.55 to 1.22 if treatment was initiated at 0 to 90 minutes and 271 to 360 minutes, respectively.[11] These results were further supported by a subsequent analysis that used additional data from the ECASS III and Echoplanar Imaging Thrombolytic Evaluation Trial (EPITHET) trials.[17] Another pooled analysis from 6 trials showed that the number needed to treat increased from 3.6 to 19.3 if treatment was initiated between 0 and 90 minutes and 271 and 360 minutes, respectively.[19] Similar results were obtained from a historical prospective cohort of a statewide registry in Germany.[20] Data from 58,353 patients treated with tPA within 4.5 hours shows that earlier administration, in increments of 15 minutes, was associated not only with decreased mortality and SICH but also with increased chance of ambulation at discharge and discharge to home.[21]

AMERICAN HEART ASSOCIATION/AMERICAN STROKE ASSOCIATION GUIDELINES

In an effort to increase the number of patients eligible for treatment, the guidelines for early management of acute stroke published in 2013[22] modified some of the initial contraindications for IV tPA published in the 2007 guidelines[23] into *relative* contraindications (**Table 1**). For example, although the FDA did not approve tPA administration within 3.0 to 4.5 hours, after publication of the ECASS III trial results, the American Heart Association/American Stroke Association (AHA/ASA) issued a Class 1, level of evidence B, recommendation for thrombolysis within the 3.0-hour to 4.5-hour window. The exclusion criteria were similar to the 3-hour window except for age older than 80 years, large stroke (National Institutes of Health Stroke Scale [NIHSS] >25), the combination of diabetes mellitus and previous stroke, and recent use of anticoagulant medication regardless of international normalized ratio (INR).[24] This recommendation was incorporated into the 2013 guidelines for treatment of acute ischemic stroke. The same guidelines empower the vascular neurologists to determine on a case-by-case basis if administration of tPA with one or more relative contraindications may be beneficial.

AREAS OF CONTROVERSY
Off-Label Use of Tissue Plasminogen Activator

The European Stroke Organization (ESO) guidelines for thrombolysis are more restrictive than the AHA/ASA guidelines. Because of insufficient information regarding tPA treatment in patients excluded from the NINDS and ECASS trials, the ESO and the European Medicines Agency do not recommend administration in these patients.[25] In a retrospective analysis of 985 Finnish patients with acute ischemic stroke, 499

Table 1
Comparison of contraindications for tPA among NINDS, ECASS II and III, and 2007 and 2013 ASA guidelines

Contraindications	NINDS	ECASS II, III	ASA 2007	ASA 2013
Age >80 y	–	+	–	–
Age <18 y	+	+	–	–
Time of onset unknown	+	+	+	+
Time of onset within 3.0–4.5 h	+	–	+	+/–
Time of onset within 4.5–6.0 h	+	–	+	+
Symptoms suggestive of subarachnoid hemorrhage	+	+	+	+
History of aneurysmal subarachnoid hemorrhage	+	–	+	+
History of intracranial hemorrhage	+	+	+	+
Intracranial neoplasm	–	–	–	+
Intracranial AVM or aneurysm	–	–	–	+
Severe head trauma	+ <3 mo	+ <2 wk[a] + <3 mo[b]	+	+
Recent intracranial or spinal surgery within 3 mo	+	+	+	+
Stroke in previous 3 mo	+	+[b]	+	+
Stroke and DM	–	+[b]	–	+[b]
Arterial puncture at a noncompressible site in the previous 7 d	+		+	+
Uncontrolled HTN (systolic >185 mm Hg and diastolic >110 mm Hg)	+	+	+	+
Intravenous/aggressive treatment of HTN	+	+[b]	–	+
Active bleeding or acute trauma (fracture) on examination		+	+	+
Blood glucose <50 mg/dL	+	+	+	+
Blood glucose >400 mg/dL	+	+	NA	NA
Warfarin with INR <1.7	+	+[b]	–	–
Warfarin with INR >1.7	+	+	+	+
If receiving heparin in previous 48 h, aPTT > normal range	+	+	+	+

Platelet count <100,000/mm³	+	+	+	NA	+
Current use of direct thrombin inhibitors or direct factor Xa inhibitors with elevated sensitive tests: aPTT, INR, PLT, ECT, TT, or factor Xa activity assays	+	NA	NA	NA	+
CT shows multilobar infarction (hypodensity >1/3 cerebral hemisphere)	+	+	+	+	+
Major early infarct signs (eg, severe edema, mass effect, midline shift)	−	+>1/3 MCA	NA	NA	−
Major deficits (NIHSS >22)	−	+ NIHSS >25	+/−	+	−
Minor, isolated, or rapidly improving stroke symptoms	+	+	+	+	+/−
Myocardial infarction in the previous 3 mo	−	−	+	+	+/−
Gastrointestinal or urinary tract hemorrhage in previous 21 d	+	+	+	+	+/−
Major surgery	+ <2 wk	+ <3 mo	+	+	+/−
Seizure with postictal residual neurologic impairments	+ at onset	+ <6 mo[a] + at onset[b]	+	+	+/−
Pregnancy	+	+[a]	+	NA	+/−
Delivery	+	+<30 d[a]	+	NA	NA
Lactation	+	+[a]	+	NA	NA

Abbreviations: +, absolute contraindication; +/−, relative contraindication; −, no contraindication; aPTT, activated partial thromboplastin time; ASA, American Stroke Association; AVM, arteriovenous malformation; CT, computed tomography; DM, diabetes mellitus; ECASS, European Cooperative Acute Stroke Study; ECT, ecarin clotting time; HTN, hypertension; INR, international normalized ratio; MCA, middle cerebral artery; NA, not addressed; NIHSS, National Institutes of Health Stroke Scale; NINDS, National Institute of Neurological Disorders and Stroke; PLT, platelets; TT, thrombin clotting time.
[a] ECASS II.
[b] ECASS III.
Data from Refs.[1,9,13,22,23]

(51%) were treated off-label. The most common reasons were age older than 80 years, mild stroke (NIHSS <5), use of IV antihypertensive agents, symptom-to-treatment longer than 3 hours, blood pressure higher than 185/110 mm Hg, and oral anticoagulation. None of these contraindications increased the risk of SICH. Only age older than 80 years predicted poor outcome.[26] Similar proportions of SICH, 3-month functional outcome, and mortality rate were seen in both on-label and off-label groups.[27] These findings were confirmed in patients who received tPA up to 4.5 hours of symptoms onset.[28] A larger retrospective analysis of a trials database including 2755 patients showed a broad trend of more favorable 3-month outcome (expressed as odds ratio [OR]) associated with tPA versus placebo in the following subgroups: 1.40 in patients older than 80, 1.50 in patients with previous stroke and diabetes mellitus, 1.42 in patients taking 1 antiplatelet agent, 2.20 in patients on Coumadin and INR of 1.7 or lower, 1.50 in patients with baseline glucose higher than 180 mg/mL, and 1.57 in patients with pretreatment NIHSS greater than 22.[29] In a prospectively collected database of 500 thrombolysed patients, no off-label criteria for tPA decreased the rate of major neurologic improvement (decrease in NIHSS >8 points) compared with on-label thrombolysis.[30] Recent data from Get With The Guidelines (GWTG) demonstrate that of 4910 patients treated within the 3.0-hour to 4.5-hour window, 1544 had at least one additional exclusion criterion. For each additional exclusion criterion, there was no increased risk of SICH or worse outcome compared with the 0 to 3-hour window.[3]

Wake-Up Stroke or Unknown Time of Onset

Treatment of wake-up stroke (WUS) is challenging because of unknown time of onset, a contraindication for tPA. In a large population-based study of 1854 patients with stroke, 14.3% were WUS. WUS had similar clinical features and outcomes with all other strokes.[31] A prospective database comparing WUS within 3 hours of symptom awareness with patients with stroke treated with tPA within the 4.5-hour window showed similar proportion of early ischemic changes. However, thrombolysed patients had better outcome (OR 2.12; 95% confidence interval [CI] 1.05–4.28; $P = .037$). Administration of tPA and baseline NIHSS were the only predictors of outcome.[32]

In a retrospective analysis of patients with WUS, tPA improved the rate of excellent and favorable outcome, at the cost of higher mortality. Compared with treatment within 3 hours of onset, thrombolysis of WUS led to similar functional outcome and safety.[33] A much larger dataset from the IST-3 comprising 17,398 patients, of whom 29.6% had WUS, showed similar functional outcome and mortality between patients with WUS and those who had stroke while awake.[34]

The use of imaging to determine the time of onset of WUS could help select the patients who might benefit from tPA. Patients with WUS with no or early ischemic changes, less than one-third of the middle cerebral artery (MCA) territory on computed tomography (CT) of the head, had similar risk of SICH and benefit from tPA as those presenting within 4.5 hours.[35] However, a perfusion CT protocol used in selection of patients with WUS or unknown last well failed to improve patients' outcome after thrombolysis.[36] Conversely, mismatch between presence of a lesion in DWI but absent on fluid attenuated inversion recovery sequence on brain MRI, helps select the patients within the 4.5-hour window[37,38] and may improve the functional status.[39–42]

Age

Age younger than 18 or older than 80 years was not a contraindication for tPA according to the AHA/ASA guidelines. However, because these patients were excluded from the ECASS trials, in the European Union, tPA was not approved in these age groups.[25] In the United States, between 2000 and 2003, 46 children were treated with tPA. They were less likely to be discharged home and had higher rate of death and dependency.[43] A MEDLINE and EMBASE search found 17 children treated for stroke, of whom 6 received IV tPA. Sixteen (94%) children survived and 12 (71%) had good outcome (modified Rankin Scale [mRS] = 0–1).[44] Although used, the role of tPA in children with stroke is not yet clearly established.

The risk of stroke increases with age; however, patients older than 80 were excluded from the ECASS and ATLANTIS trials, but not from NINDS or IST-3. In several studies, although there was no increase in SICH after IV tPA, outcome was worse in patients older than 80 compared with those younger.[45–49] In another study of 77 consecutive patients treated with tPA within 4.5 hours, age older than 80 years was an independent risk factor for SICH and death at 3 months but was not associated with functional outcome.[50] In a systematic review of 6 studies with 2244 patients treated with tPA, patients 80 years or older had a mortality rate 3 times higher and a reduced chance of favorable outcome compared with younger patients.[51] In IST-3, tPA given within 6 hours did not reduce mortality or disability, but an ordinal analysis showed a significant shift in disability score in elderly patients. Most patients treated within 3 hours were older than 80 years, and the benefit of tPA was as large as in younger patients.[15] In 2008, the ESO's updated guidelines suggest treatment with tPA within 3 hours of selected patients younger than 18 years and older than 80 years, acknowledging that this is an off-label recommendation.[52] Recent data from GWTG has shown that patients older than 80 years do not have worse outcome if treated within the 3.0-hour to 4.5-hour window compared with the 0 to 3-hour window.[3] Thrombolysis may be considered in patients older than 80 years up to 4.5 hours from stroke onset if no other contraindications exist.

Recent Cerebral Infarction

In a case series, 3 of 6 patients with recent stroke, 6 days to 10 weeks before, who were treated with tPA had asymptomatic petechial ICH.[53] It is not clear how recent a cerebral infarct must be for it to be safe to give IV tPA.

History of Intracerebral Hemorrhage

Given that history of ICH continues to be a contraindication for tPA, insufficient data exist in patients with previous symptomatic ICH. A study of risk of ICH in patients with previous cerebral microbleeds (CMBs) on MRI included 326 patients. Frequency of symptomatic hemorrhage/parenchymal hematoma increased from 1.2%/5.7% in patients without CMBs to 30.0%/30.0% in patients with 5 or more CMBs, respectively.[54] In another retrospective analysis, CMBs detected on pretreatment susceptibility-weighted MRI did not increase the risk for ICH or worsen outcome.[55] The impact of previous CMBs on outcome of stroke treated with tPA is still unknown.

Coagulopathy

Any coagulopathy leading to bleeding tendency is a major contraindication for thrombolysis. The rate of unsuspected coagulopathy was 0.4% in a retrospective analysis of 470 patients, supporting the current policy of initiation of thrombolysis *before the coagulation studies become available*.[56]

The NINDS tPA Stroke Trial did not find aspirin to increase the risk of SICH or improve outcome. Data from a single-center prospective observational cohort study showed that antiplatelet medication used before thrombolysis was associated with greater benefit (OR 2.0) in spite of a higher incidence of SICH (OR 6.0).[57] In retrospective analysis of tPA given within 3 hours, no correlation was found between previous antiplatelet use and SICH, recanalization rate, or good outcome.[58] Analysis of a large registry found no significant difference in the rate of SICH, or 7-day or 90-day mortalities between the groups on aspirin alone and on no antiplatelet treatment. However, dual antiplatelet treatment before tPA use was associated with a higher rate of SICH (14.3% per SITS–MOST or 21.4% per ECASS II definitions).[59]

Although not a formal contraindication for tPA within 3 hours, pretreatment with Coumadin and INR less than 1.7 were found to be associated with an increased risk of SICH in 2 small retrospective studies of thrombolysed patients.[60,61] Data from the larger Registry of the Canadian Stroke Network and SITS-ISTR did not confirm this concern.[62,63] In a historical prospective study from the Cleveland area of 70 patients who received tPA, the most frequent protocol violation, in 37.1% of patients, was administration of antiplatelet agents or anticoagulants within 24 hours of tPA administration. Although the rate of SICH and mortality in these patients was significantly increased, 15.7% and 15.7% respectively, concomitant use of antiplatelets or anticoagulation was not associated with these outcomes ($P>.99$).[64] In a larger study of 499 thrombolysed patients, none of the 5 patients who were taking oral anticoagulant with INR greater than 1.7, low molecular weight heparin, or IV heparin with elevated activated partial thromboplastin time (aPTT) died. Thrombocytopenia was found in 0.7% of patients and did not increase the risk of SICH.[26] Any baseline coagulopathy was found in 36 (5%) of 688 patients who received tPA, but it was not associated with a higher SICH or mortality.[65] The ECASS III trial excluded patients on anticoagulation with normal coagulation profile. However, data from GWTG does not demonstrate worse outcome in these patients treated within the 3.0-hour to 4.5-hour window compared with those treated within 0 to 3 hours.[3]

According to the current guidelines, the direct thrombin inhibitors and direct factor Xa inhibitors taken within 48 hours represent a contraindication for tPA unless the following tests are normal: PTT, INR, platelet count, ecarin clotting time (ECT), thrombin time (TT), or the appropriate direct factor X activity assay. However, the new anticoagulants may have a reduced risk of ICH compared with warfarin.[66] Thrombolysis administered during treatment with dabigatran was safe in several patients in whom PTT was normal.[67–72] One fatal ICH after tPA administration in a patient with normal PTT, who took dabigatran 3 hours earlier, suggests caution against reliance on this test alone when deciding about thrombolysis,[73] because PTT may be normal despite a prolonged TT.[74] Case reports of safety of thrombolysis in patients taking rivaroxaban and apixaban were also published.[75–81] Because of the small number of patients with coagulopathy who received tPA safely, administration of tPA in this category of patients cannot be recommended at this time.

Uncontrolled Hypertension

Uncontrolled hypertension remains a contraindication for tPA. In the NINDS trial, patients treated with tPA had worse outcome if their postrandomization blood pressure (BP) was higher than 180/105 mm Hg and needed treatment than if they were still hypertensive but did not require treatment.[82]

Protocol violations of BP management before thrombolysis were more frequent in patients with SICH than without (26% vs 12%; $P = .019$) and led to increased risk of SICH (OR 2.59; 95% CI 1.07–6.25; $P = .034$).[83] Data from the SITS-ISTR demonstrated that systolic BP higher than 180 mm Hg after thrombolysis is associated with worse outcome. There is a linear association with SICH, as well as a U-shaped association with mortality and independence. The most favorable systolic BP range was from 141 to 150 mm Hg.[84] However, after controlling for more variables recorded in a single-center registry of 985 patients who received thrombolysis, no association between SICH and elevated BP was found. Also, use of IV antihypertensive medication before thrombolysis was not associated with poor outcome.[26]

Severe or Large Stroke

The 3 ECASS thrombolysis trials excluded patients with NIHSS greater than 25 or radiological signs of large stroke (diffuse cerebral edema, parenchymal hypoattenuation, or effacement of sulci greater than one-third of the MCA territory).[8,9,13] In the NINDS trial, higher NIHSS, brain edema (acute hypodensity), and mass effect on CT before treatment were the only variables independently associated with an increased risk of SICH; nevertheless, tPA increased the chance of favorable outcome at 3 months.[85] Subgroup analysis of the same trial shows that stroke severity did not alter the likelihood of responding favorably to tPA.[86] Data from GWTG shows that patients with NIHSS greater than 25 did not have worse outcome if tPA was given within the window of 0 to 3.0 hours or 3.0 to 4.5 hours.[3] This suggests that tPA may be considered in patients with large stroke up to 4.5 hours from symptoms onset.

Presence of Cerebral Vascular Malformations

Several retrospective reviews have demonstrated similar safety and benefit of thrombolysis in patients with and without unruptured aneurysms.[87–89] Diagnosis of cerebral cavernous malformation was not associated with a raise in the risk of SICH in 9 patients who underwent thrombolysis.[90] In a case series of 15 patients with acute stroke evaluated with early CT angiography there was one incidental aneurysm that eventually ruptured even without tPA administration, suggesting caution when considering tPA in patients with known aneurysm.[91]

Tumors with or Without Metastatic Lesions to Brain

In a nationwide inpatient sample of 32,576 thrombolysed patients, the patients with stroke with any cancer and those without had similar rates of home discharge, inpatient mortality, or ICH. Subgroup analysis showed that after tPA, solid tumors had worse in-hospital mortality and home discharge than liquid tumors. Metastatic cancer had the worst prognosis, but was not associated with a higher risk of ICH.[92]

Mild Stroke or Rapidly Improving Symptoms: Too Good to Treat

The patients who presented with "minor or rapidly improving symptoms" were excluded from the NINDS trials.[1] Prespecified definitions of "minor" were isolated dysarthria, isolated facial weakness, isolated ataxia, or isolated sensory loss. Rapidly improving symptoms were excluded to avoid treating transient ischemic attacks.[93] In subsequent studies, favorable outcome was achieved in 80% of untreated patients with NIHSS 0 or 1 if on the items of level of consciousness, gaze, facial palsy, or sensory or dysarthria.[94,95]

Between 2% and 28% of patients with minor stroke or rapidly improving symptoms not treated with tPA had poor outcome.[95–98] The initial severity of stroke is the major predictor for poor outcome (mRS >2).[99] In one study, the patients who improved by NIHSS greater than 4 points before tPA was withheld were more likely to experience subsequent worsening.[97] Fluctuating neurologic symptoms by 4 points or more on the NIHSS portend a high risk of stroke.[100] In a prospective study, fluctuations ceased after thrombolysis and all patients had favorable outcome (mRS = 0–2) at 3 months.[101] In patients with clinical symptoms and decreased perfusion but no lesion in DWI on MRI, tPA reversed all the symptoms.[102] Benefit of tPA along the entire age range was seen in a large prospective registry including 54,917 patients, of which 890 patients had NIHSS of 5 or less.[103] In a meta-analysis of 8 studies, the association of tPA with good outcome (mRS = 0–1) in patients with minor stroke just reached statistical significance (pooled OR 1.319; P = .047), without increase in mortality.[104]

Criteria have been proposed by an expert panel (The REexamining Acute Eligibility for Thrombolysis [TREAT] Task Force) to help clinicians evaluate patients with rapid improvement. The panel recommends treatment for all patients who rapidly improve but are still left with any of the following deficits: complete hemianopsia, severe aphasia, visual or sensory extinction, any weakness limiting sustained effort against gravity, any cumulative deficits leading to a total NIHSS of greater than 5, or any remaining, but potentially disabling deficit in the view of the patient and the physician.[93] An open discussion with the patient and clinical judgment are required.

Recent Acute Myocardial Infarction

Patients with acute myocardial infarction (AMI) were excluded in the NINDS trials to avoid treatment of simultaneous thrombi in the coronary and cerebral vessels, a situation that may have reduced the efficacy of tPA, especially considering that the dose for acute stroke is lower than for AMI. Thrombolysis is contraindicated in patients with acute non–ST-elevation MI (NSTEMI) because of lack of benefit and increased risk of fatal and nonfatal MI. Instead, anticoagulation with heparin is recommended for NSTEMI, a treatment currently discouraged in patients with stroke. Thrombolysis with tPA may be used for acute ST-elevation MI (STEMI) if percutaneous coronary intervention is not available within 90 minutes from symptom onset.[105,106] For STEMI, the tPA dose is higher (1.1 mg/kg), infusion protocol may be accelerated, and the therapeutic window is longer (12 hours) than for stroke. Because of these considerations, the best course of treatment for patients with stroke and AMI with or without ST-elevation remains to be determined. Also unknown is how soon after stabilization of AMI is it safe to administer tPA. Therefore, recent AMI is a relative contraindication for tPA.

Gastrointestinal and Urinary Tract Hemorrhage Within 21 Days

Most gastrointestinal and urinary tract (GI/U) wound healing occurs within 21 days, after which a plateau is seen in regaining of the tensile strength, which does not return to baseline however.[107] Because tPA use has been avoided in these patients, it is not known when the earliest time is that tPA can be given safely. Clinicians must weigh the potential risks of severe GI/U hemorrhage and transfusions with potential benefit of reduction of severity and disability of the stroke. The balance may depend on the stroke severity at the time of treatment and how recent and active the bleeding is or was.

Recent Major Surgery

A retrospective review of 17 patients treated within 3 weeks of surgery[108] supports the observation from several case reports that, in selected patients, tPA may be used after major surgery.[109–111] The potential for hemorrhagic complications and their management should be considered individually.

Hyperglycemia

Hyperglycemia in nondiabetic patients with acute stroke is more than a stress reaction; it is also associated with increased mortality.[112] Hyperglycemia and diabetes mellitus in patients treated with thrombolysis were independent predictors of ICH.[113] In a prospective study, the risk of SICH increased linearly to blood glucose level, and was associated with increased risk of death or disability at 3 months.[114] The combination of history of stroke and diabetes was the only off-label criterion associated with increased rate of neurologic deterioration (increase in NIHSS >4 points).[30] This was not seen in a recent review of "GWTG" patients treated in the United States

Table 2
Recommendation for thrombolysis with tPA in different clinical and laboratory scenarios

Clinical or Laboratory Condition	Recommendation for IV tPA	Level of Evidence
Age >80 y	+	T1
Age <18 y	+/−	T4
Time of onset unknown	−	T1
Time of onset within 3.0–4.5 h	+/−[a]	T1
Time of onset within 4.5–6.0 h	−	T1
Symptoms suggestive of subarachnoid hemorrhage	−	T4
History of aneurysmal subarachnoid hemorrhage	−	T4
History of intracranial hemorrhage	−	T4
Intracranial neoplasm	+/−	T4
Intracranial AVM or aneurysm	+/−	T4
Serious head trauma in previous 3 mo	−	T4
Recent intracranial or spinal surgery (3 mo)	−	T4
Stroke in previous 3 mo	+/−	T4
Stroke and DM within 3.0–4.5-h window	+/−	T3
Arterial puncture at a noncompressible site in the previous 7 d	−	T4
Uncontrolled HTN (systolic >185 mm Hg and diastolic >110 mm Hg)	−	T3
IV/aggressive treatment of HTN	+	T2
Active bleeding or acute trauma (fracture) on examination	−	T4
Blood glucose <50 mg/dL	−	T4
Blood glucose >400 mg/dL	+/−	T3
Warfarin with INR <1.7	+	T1
Warfarin with INR >1.7	−	T4
If receiving heparin in previous 48 h, aPTT > normal range	−	T4
Platelet count <100,000 mm^3	−	T4
Current use of direct thrombin inhibitors or direct factor Xa inhibitors with elevated sensitive tests: aPTT, INR, PLT, ECT, TT, or factor Xa activity assays)	−	T4
CT shows multilobar infarction (hypodensity >1/3 cerebral hemisphere)	−	T4
Major early infarct signs (eg, severe edema, mass effect, midline shift)	+	T2
Major deficits (NIHSS >25) within 0–3-h window	+	T2
Major deficits (NIHSS >25) within 3.0–4.5-h window	+/−	T3
Minor, isolated, or rapidly improving stroke symptoms	+	T2
Myocardial infarction in the previous 3 mo	+/−	T4
Gastrointestinal or urinary tract hemorrhage in previous 21 d	+/−	T4
Major surgery within 14 days	+/−	T4
Seizure with postictal residual neurologic impairments	+/−	T4
Pregnancy	+/−	T4

Abbreviations: +, recommended; +/−, may be considered; −, not recommended; aPTT, activated partial thromboplastin time; AVM, arteriovenous malformation; DM, diabetes mellitus; ECT, ecarin clotting time; HTN, hypertension; INR, international normalized ratio; IV, intravenous; NIHSS, National Institutes of Health Stroke Scale; PLT, platelets; tPA, tissue plasminogen activator; TT, thrombin time.

[a] Recommended in accordance with the American Heart Association/American Stroke Association and European Stroke Organization guidelines and reasonable to consider in patients older than 80 years, with history of both DM and stroke, NIHSS >25 and use of Coumadin, and INR ≤1.7; T1–T4 categories.

from 3.0 to 4.5 hours. These patients still do better with tPA that without tPA.[3] It is reasonable to treat hyperglycemia as early as possible; however, if intensive treatment is associated with improved outcome, it will be determined by a clinical trial currently enrolling patients.[115]

Seizures

Seizures are one of the most common mimics of stroke[116–119] in which thrombolysis was found to be safe.[120] Distinguishing a postictal state from stroke may be challenging when confusion or aphasia are present. CT perfusion may show hypoperfusion in the area of ischemia[36] that is similar in the postictal state[121] if not confirmed by vessel occlusion.[122] It is reasonable to consider treatment if the seizure appears to be associated with or triggered by an infarct.

Pregnancy and Menstruation

Pregnancy was excluded from the stroke clinical trials and is a relative contraindication for IV tPA.[22] Selected pregnant patients with stroke were treated with tPA successfully.[123–126] Two pregnant women had massive subchorionic hematoma, one of which resolved spontaneously.[127] Miscarriage has been reported.[128] Thrombolysis was used successfully in several menstruating women with stroke without increased risk of bleeding, although blood transfusion may be needed.[129]

SUMMARY

For most contraindications to tPA, there are no randomized clinical trials. Nevertheless, there is mounting evidence suggesting that patients with acute ischemic stroke may still benefit from thrombolysis despite the presence of some contraindications. The level of evidence evolves as more information is gathered. Some of the previous contraindications presented here have been incorporated in the current guidelines and are no longer considered as such. Details of the levels of evidence of clinical efficacy of therapeutic intervention used are modified from the National Stroke Association guidelines for the management of transient ischemic attacks.[130]

Table 2 details recommendation for thrombolysis in different clinical and laboratory conditions. A more rigorous evaluation of the outcome of patients with acute stroke treated with tPA despite the presence of contraindications should be the focus of future research.

REFERENCES

1. Tissue plasminogen activator for acute ischemic stroke. The National Institute of Neurological Disorders and Stroke rt-PA Stroke study group. N Engl J Med 1995;333(24):1581–7.
2. Adeoye O, Hornung R, Khatri P, et al. Recombinant tissue-type plasminogen activator use for ischemic stroke in the United States: a doubling of treatment rates over the course of 5 years. Stroke 2011;42(7):1952–5.
3. Cronin CA, Sheth KN, Zhao X, et al. Adherence to third European cooperative acute stroke study 3- to 4.5-hour exclusions and association with outcome: data from get with the guidelines-stroke. Stroke 2014;45(9):2745–9.
4. Balami JS, Hadley G, Sutherland BA, et al. The exact science of stroke thrombolysis and the quiet art of patient selection. Brain 2013;136(Pt 12):3528–53.
5. O'Connor RE, McGraw P, Edelsohn L. Thrombolytic therapy for acute ischemic stroke: why the majority of patients remain ineligible for treatment. Ann Emerg Med 1999;33(1):9–14.

6. Barber PA, Zhang J, Demchuk AM, et al. Why are stroke patients excluded from TPA therapy? An analysis of patient eligibility. Neurology 2001;56(8): 1015–20.

7. Hills NK, Johnston SC. Why are eligible thrombolysis candidates left untreated? Am J Prev Med 2006;31(6 Suppl 2):S210–6.

8. Hacke W, Kaste M, Fieschi C, et al. Intravenous thrombolysis with recombinant tissue plasminogen activator for acute hemispheric stroke. The European Cooperative Acute Stroke Study (ECASS). JAMA 1995;274(13):1017–25.

9. Hacke W, Kaste M, Fieschi C, et al. Randomised double-blind placebo-controlled trial of thrombolytic therapy with intravenous alteplase in acute ischaemic stroke (ECASS II). Second European-Australasian Acute Stroke Study Investigators. Lancet 1998;352(9136):1245–51.

10. Clark WM, Wissman S, Albers GW, et al. Recombinant tissue-type plasminogen activator (Alteplase) for ischemic stroke 3 to 5 hours after symptom onset. The ATLANTIS study: a randomized controlled trial. Alteplase thrombolysis for acute noninterventional therapy in ischemic stroke. JAMA 1999;282(21): 2019–26.

11. Hacke W, Donnan G, Fieschi C, et al. Association of outcome with early stroke treatment: pooled analysis of ATLANTIS, ECASS, and NINDS rt-PA stroke trials. Lancet 2004;363(9411):768–74.

12. Davis SM, Donnan GA, Parsons MW, et al. Effects of alteplase beyond 3 h after stroke in the Echoplanar Imaging Thrombolytic Evaluation Trial (EPITHET): a placebo-controlled randomised trial. Lancet Neurol 2008;7(4):299–309.

13. Hacke W, Kaste M, Bluhmki E, et al. Thrombolysis with alteplase 3 to 4.5 hours after acute ischemic stroke. N Engl J Med 2008;359(13):1317–29.

14. Wahlgren N, Ahmed N, Davalos A, et al. Thrombolysis with alteplase 3–4.5 h after acute ischaemic stroke (SITS-ISTR): an observational study. Lancet 2008; 372(9646):1303–9.

15. IST-3 Collaborative Group, Sandercock P, Wardlaw JM, et al. The benefits and harms of intravenous thrombolysis with recombinant tissue plasminogen activator within 6 h of acute ischaemic stroke (the third International Stroke Trial [IST-3]): a randomised controlled trial. Lancet 2012;379(9834):2352–63.

16. IST-3 Collaborative Group. Effect of thrombolysis with alteplase within 6 h of acute ischaemic stroke on long-term outcomes (the third International Stroke Trial [IST-3]): 18-month follow-up of a randomised controlled trial. Lancet Neurol 2013;12(8):768–76.

17. Lees KR, Bluhmki E, von Kummer R, et al. Time to treatment with intravenous alteplase and outcome in stroke: an updated pooled analysis of ECASS, ATLANTIS, NINDS, and EPITHET trials. Lancet 2010;375(9727):1695–703.

18. de Los Ríos la Rosa F, Khoury J, Kissela BM, et al. Eligibility for intravenous recombinant tissue-type plasminogen activator within a population: the effect of the European Cooperative Acute Stroke Study (ECASS) III trial. Stroke 2012; 43(6):1591–5.

19. Lansberg MG, Schrooten M, Bluhmki E, et al. Treatment time-specific number needed to treat estimates for tissue plasminogen activator therapy in acute stroke based on shifts over the entire range of the modified Rankin Scale. Stroke 2009;40(6):2079–84.

20. Gumbinger C, Reuter B, Stock C, et al. Time to treatment with recombinant tissue plasminogen activator and outcome of stroke in clinical practice: retrospective analysis of hospital quality assurance data with comparison with results from randomised clinical trials. BMJ 2014;348:g3429.

21. Saver JL, Fonarow GC, Smith EE, et al. Time to treatment with intravenous tissue plasminogen activator and outcome from acute ischemic stroke. JAMA 2013; 309(23):2480–8.

22. Jauch EC, Saver JL, Adams HP Jr, et al. Guidelines for the early management of patients with acute ischemic stroke: a guideline for healthcare professionals from the American Heart Association/American Stroke Association. Stroke 2013;44(3):870–947.

23. Adams HP Jr, del Zoppo G, Alberts MJ, et al. Guidelines for the early management of adults with ischemic stroke: a guideline from the American Heart Association/American Stroke Association Stroke Council, Clinical Cardiology Council, Cardiovascular Radiology and Intervention Council, and the Atherosclerotic Peripheral Vascular Disease and Quality of Care Outcomes in Research Interdisciplinary Working Groups: the American Academy of Neurology affirms the value of this guideline as an educational tool for neurologists. Stroke 2007;38(5): 1655–711.

24. Del Zoppo GJ, Saver JL, American Heart Association Stroke Council, et al. Expansion of the time window for treatment of acute ischemic stroke with intravenous tissue plasminogen activator: a science advisory from the American Heart Association/American Stroke Association. Stroke 2009;40(8):2945–8.

25. European Stroke Organisation Executive Committee, ESO Writing Committee. Guidelines for management of ischaemic stroke and transient ischaemic attack 2008. Cerebrovasc Dis 2008;25(5):457–507.

26. Meretoja A, Putaala J, Tatlisumak T, et al. Off-label thrombolysis is not associated with poor outcome in patients with stroke. Stroke 2010;41(7):1450–8.

27. Guillan M, Alonso-Canovas A, Garcia-Caldentey J, et al. Off-label intravenous thrombolysis in acute stroke. Eur J Neurol 2012;19(3):390–4.

28. Kvistad CE, Logallo N, Thomassen L, et al. Safety of off-label stroke treatment with tissue plasminogen activator. Acta Neurol Scand 2013;128(1):48–53.

29. Frank B, Grotta JC, Alexandrov AV, et al. Thrombolysis in stroke despite contraindications or warnings? Stroke 2013;44(3):727–33.

30. Cappellari M, Moretto G, Micheletti N, et al. Off-label thrombolysis versus full adherence to the current European Alteplase license: impact on early clinical outcomes after acute ischemic stroke. J Thromb Thrombolysis 2014;37(4): 549–56.

31. Mackey J, Kleindorfer D, Sucharew H, et al. Population-based study of wake-up strokes. Neurology 2011;76(19):1662–7.

32. Roveri L, La Gioia S, Ghidinelli C, et al. Wake-up stroke within 3 hours of symptom awareness: imaging and clinical features compared to standard recombinant tissue plasminogen activator treated stroke. J Stroke Cerebrovasc Dis 2013;22(6):703–8.

33. Barreto AD, Martin-Schild S, Hallevi H, et al. Thrombolytic therapy for patients who wake-up with stroke. Stroke 2009;40(3):827–32.

34. Moradiya Y, Janjua N. Presentation and outcomes of "wake-up strokes" in a large randomized stroke trial: analysis of data from the International Stroke Trial. J Stroke Cerebrovasc Dis 2013;22(8):e286–92.

35. Manawadu D, Bodla S, Jarosz J, et al. A case-controlled comparison of thrombolysis outcomes between wake-up and known time of onset ischemic stroke patients. Stroke 2013;44(8):2226–31.

36. Cortijo E, Calleja AI, Garcia-Bermejo P, et al. Perfusion computed tomography makes it possible to overcome important SITS-MOST exclusion criteria for the endovenous thrombolysis of cerebral infarction. Rev Neurol 2012;54(5):271–6.

37. Aoki J, Kimura K, Iguchi Y, et al. FLAIR can estimate the onset time in acute ischemic stroke patients. J Neurol Sci 2010;293(1–2):39–44.
38. Thomalla G, Cheng B, Ebinger M, et al. DWI-FLAIR mismatch for the identification of patients with acute ischaemic stroke within 4.5 h of symptom onset (PRE-FLAIR): a multicentre observational study. Lancet Neurol 2011;10(11):978–86.
39. Breuer L, Schellinger PD, Huttner HB, et al. Feasibility and safety of magnetic resonance imaging-based thrombolysis in patients with stroke on awakening: initial single-centre experience. Int J Stroke 2010;5(2):68–73.
40. Aoki J, Kimura K, Iguchi Y, et al. Intravenous thrombolysis based on diffusion-weighted imaging and fluid-attenuated inversion recovery mismatch in acute stroke patients with unknown onset time. Cerebrovasc Dis 2011;31(5):435–41.
41. Manawadu D, Bodla S, Keep J, et al. An observational study of thrombolysis outcomes in wake-up ischemic stroke patients. Stroke 2013;44(2):427–31.
42. Bai Q, Zhao Z, Fu P, et al. Clinical outcomes of fast MRI-based thrombolysis in wake-up strokes compared to superacute ischemic strokes within 12 hours. Neurol Res 2013;35(5):492–7.
43. Janjua N, Nasar A, Lynch JK, et al. Thrombolysis for ischemic stroke in children: data from the nationwide inpatient sample. Stroke 2007;38(6):1850–4.
44. Arnold M, Steinlin M, Baumann A, et al. Thrombolysis in childhood stroke: report of 2 cases and review of the literature. Stroke 2009;40(3):801–7.
45. Berrouschot J, Röther J, Glahn J, et al. Outcome and severe hemorrhagic complications of intravenous thrombolysis with tissue plasminogen activator in very old (> or = 80 years) stroke patients. Stroke 2005;36(11):2421–5.
46. Bhatnagar P, Sinha D, Parker RA, et al. Intravenous thrombolysis in acute ischaemic stroke: a systematic review and meta-analysis to aid decision making in patients over 80 years of age. J Neurol Neurosurg Psychiatr 2011;82(7):712–7.
47. Boulouis G, Dumont F, Cordonnier C, et al. Intravenous thrombolysis for acute cerebral ischaemia in old stroke patients ≥ 80 years of age. J Neurol 2012;259(7):1461–7.
48. Bray BD, Campbell J, Hoffman A, et al. Stroke thrombolysis in England: an age stratified analysis of practice and outcome. Age Ageing 2013;42(2):240–5.
49. Sylaja PN, Cote R, Buchan AM, et al. Investigators CAfSESC. Thrombolysis in patients older than 80 years with acute ischaemic stroke: Canadian Alteplase for Stroke Effectiveness Study. J Neurol Neurosurg Psychiatr 2006;77(7):826–9.
50. Henriksen EH, Ljøstad U, Tveiten A, et al. TPA for ischemic stroke in patients ≥80 years. Acta Neurol Scand 2013;127(5):309–15.
51. Engelter ST, Bonati LH, Lyrer PA. Intravenous thrombolysis in stroke patients of > or = 80 versus < 80 years of age—a systematic review across cohort studies. Age Ageing 2006;35(6):572–80.
52. European Stroke Organization (ESO). Karolinska Stroke Update 2008, Final draft per 20081118, ESO GC Statement on revised guidelines for intravenous thrombolysis. Available at: http://www.congrex-switzerland.com/fileadmin/files/2013/eso-stroke/pdf/ESO_Guideline_Update_Jan_2009.pdf. Accessed November 14, 2014.
53. Alhazzaa M, Sharma M, Blacquiere D, et al. Thrombolysis despite recent stroke: a case series. Stroke 2013;44(6):1736–8.
54. Dannenberg S, Scheitz JF, Rozanski M, et al. Number of cerebral microbleeds and risk of intracerebral hemorrhage after intravenous thrombolysis. Stroke 2014;45(10):2900–5.

55. Gratz PP, El-Koussy M, Hsieh K, et al. Preexisting cerebral microbleeds on susceptibility-weighted magnetic resonance imaging and post-thrombolysis bleeding risk in 392 patients. Stroke 2014;45(6):1684–8.
56. Rost NS, Masrur S, Pervez MA, et al. Unsuspected coagulopathy rarely prevents IV thrombolysis in acute ischemic stroke. Neurology 2009;73(23): 1957–62.
57. Uyttenboogaart M, Koch MW, Koopman K, et al. Safety of antiplatelet therapy prior to intravenous thrombolysis in acute ischemic stroke. Arch Neurol 2008; 65(5):607–11.
58. Ibrahim MM, Sebastian J, Hussain M, et al. Does current oral antiplatelet agent or subtherapeutic anticoagulation use have an effect on tissue-plasminogen-activator-mediated recanalization rate in patients with acute ischemic stroke? Cerebrovasc Dis 2010;30(5):508–13.
59. Pan Y, Chen Q, Liao X, et al. Preexisting dual antiplatelet treatment increases the risk of post-thrombolysis intracranial hemorrhage in Chinese stroke patients. Neurol Res 2015;37(1):64–8.
60. Prabhakaran S, Rivolta J, Vieira JR, et al. Symptomatic intracerebral hemorrhage among eligible warfarin-treated patients receiving intravenous tissue plasminogen activator for acute ischemic stroke. Arch Neurol 2010;67(5): 559–63.
61. Seet RC, Zhang Y, Moore SA, et al. Subtherapeutic international normalized ratio in warfarin-treated patients increases the risk for symptomatic intracerebral hemorrhage after intravenous thrombolysis. Stroke 2011;42(8):2333–5.
62. Vergouwen MDI, Casaubon LK, Swartz RH, et al. Subtherapeutic warfarin is not associated with increased hemorrhage rates in ischemic strokes treated with tissue plasminogen activator. Stroke 2011;42(4):1041–5.
63. Mazya MV, Lees KR, Markus R, et al. Safety of intravenous thrombolysis for ischemic stroke in patients treated with warfarin. Ann Neurol 2013;74(2): 266–74.
64. Katzan IL, Furlan AJ, Lloyd LE, et al. Use of tissue-type plasminogen activator for acute ischemic stroke: the Cleveland area experience. JAMA 2000;283(9): 1151–8.
65. Brunner F, Tomandl B, Schröter A, et al. Hemorrhagic complications after systemic thrombolysis in acute stroke patients with abnormal baseline coagulation. Eur J Neurol 2011;18(12):1407–11.
66. Pfeilschifter W, Bohmann F, Baumgarten P, et al. Thrombolysis with recombinant tissue plasminogen activator under dabigatran anticoagulation in experimental stroke. Ann Neurol 2012;71(5):624–33.
67. De Smedt A, De Raedt S, Nieboer K, et al. Intravenous thrombolysis with recombinant tissue plasminogen activator in a stroke patient treated with dabigatran. Cerebrovasc Dis 2010;30(5):533–4.
68. Marrone LC, Marrone AC. Thrombolysis in an ischemic stroke patient on dabigatran anticoagulation: a case report. Cerebrovasc Dis 2012;34(3):246–7.
69. Inaishi J, Nogawa S, Mano Y, et al. Successful thrombolysis without hemorrhage in a patient with cardioembolic stroke under dabigatran treatment—a case report and review of literature. Rinsho Shinkeigaku 2014;54(3):238–40.
70. Lee VH, Conners JJ, Prabhakaran S. Intravenous thrombolysis in a stroke patient taking dabigatran. J Stroke Cerebrovasc Dis 2012;21(8):916.e11–2.
71. Pfeilschifter W, Abruscato M, Hövelmann S, et al. Thrombolysis in a stroke patient on dabigatran anticoagulation: case report and synopsis of published cases. Case Rep Neurol 2013;5(1):56–61.

72. Diogo C, Duarte J, Sobral S, et al. Good outcome after intravenous thrombolysis for acute stroke in a patient under treatment with dabigatran. Am J Emerg Med 2014;32(11):1435.e1–2.
73. Casado Naranjo I, Portilla-Cuenca JC, Jimenez Caballero PE, et al. Fatal intracerebral hemorrhage associated with administration of recombinant tissue plasminogen activator in a stroke patient on treatment with dabigatran. Cerebrovasc Dis 2011;32(6):614–5.
74. Kate M, Szkotak A, Witt A, et al. Proposed approach to thrombolysis in dabigatran-treated patients presenting with ischemic stroke. J Stroke Cerebrovasc Dis 2014;23(6):1351–5.
75. Fluri F, Heinen F, Kleinschnitz C. Intravenous thrombolysis in a stroke patient receiving rivaroxaban. Cerebrovasc Dis Extra 2013;3(1):153–5.
76. Bornkamm K, Harloff A. Safe intravenous thrombolysis in acute stroke despite treatment with rivaroxaban. J Clin Neurosci 2014;21(11):2012–3.
77. Kawiorski MM, Alonso-Canovas A, de Felipe Mimbrera A, et al. Successful intravenous thrombolysis in acute ischaemic stroke in a patient on rivaroxaban treatment. Thromb Haemost 2014;111(3):557–8.
78. Kimura S, Ogata T, Fukae J, et al. Revascularization for acute ischemic stroke is safe for rivaroxaban users. J Stroke Cerebrovasc Dis 2014;23(9):e427–31.
79. Neal AJ, Campbell BC, Chandratheva A, et al. Intravenous thrombolysis for acute ischaemic stroke in the setting of rivaroxaban use. J Clin Neurosci 2014;21(11):2013–5.
80. Seiffge DJ, Traenka C, Gensicke H, et al. Intravenous thrombolysis in stroke patients receiving rivaroxaban. Eur J Neurol 2014;21(1):e3–4.
81. De Smedt A, Cambron M, Nieboer K, et al. Intravenous thrombolysis with recombinant tissue plasminogen activator in a stroke patient treated with apixaban. Int J Stroke 2014;9(7):E31.
82. Brott T, Lu M, Kothari R, et al. Hypertension and its treatment in the NINDS rt-PA Stroke Trial. Stroke 1998;29(8):1504–9.
83. Tsivgoulis G, Frey JL, Flaster M, et al. Pre-tissue plasminogen activator blood pressure levels and risk of symptomatic intracerebral hemorrhage. Stroke 2009;40(11):3631–4.
84. Ahmed N, Wahlgren N, Brainin M, et al. Relationship of blood pressure, antihypertensive therapy, and outcome in ischemic stroke treated with intravenous thrombolysis: retrospective analysis from Safe Implementation of Thrombolysis in Stroke-International Stroke Thrombolysis Register (SITS-ISTR). Stroke 2009;40(7):2442–9.
85. Intracerebral hemorrhage after intravenous t-PA therapy for ischemic stroke. The NINDS t-PA Stroke Study Group. Stroke 1997;28(11):2109–18.
86. Generalized efficacy of t-PA for acute stroke. Subgroup analysis of the NINDS t-PA Stroke Trial. Stroke 1997;28(11):2119–25.
87. Edwards NJ, Kamel H, Josephson SA. The safety of intravenous thrombolysis for ischemic stroke in patients with pre-existing cerebral aneurysms: a case series and review of the literature. Stroke 2012;43(2):412–6.
88. Mittal MK, Seet RC, Zhang Y, et al. Safety of intravenous thrombolysis in acute ischemic stroke patients with saccular intracranial aneurysms. J Stroke Cerebrovasc Dis 2013;22(5):639–43.
89. Kim JT, Park MS, Yoon W, et al. Detection and significance of incidental unruptured cerebral aneurysms in patients undergoing intravenous thrombolysis for acute ischemic stroke. J Neuroimaging 2012;22(2):197–200.
90. Erdur H, Scheitz JF, Tütüncü S, et al. Safety of thrombolysis in patients with acute ischemic stroke and cerebral cavernous malformations. Stroke 2014;45(6):1846–8.

91. Chuang YM, Chao AC, Teng MM, et al. Use of CT angiography in patient selection for thrombolytic therapy. Am J Emerg Med 2003;21(3):167–72.
92. Murthy SB, Karanth S, Shah S, et al. Thrombolysis for acute ischemic stroke in patients with cancer: a population study. Stroke 2013;44(12):3573–6.
93. Re-examining Acute Eligibility for Thrombolysis Task Force, Levine SR, Khatri P, et al. Review, historical context, and clarifications of the NINDS rt-PA stroke trials exclusion criteria: part 1: rapidly improving stroke symptoms. Stroke 2013;44(9): 2500–5.
94. Breuer L, Blinzler C, Huttner HB, et al. Off-label thrombolysis for acute ischemic stroke: rate, clinical outcome and safety are influenced by the definition of 'minor stroke'. Cerebrovasc Dis 2011;32(2):177–85.
95. Park TH, Hong KS, Choi JC, et al. Validation of minor stroke definitions for thrombolysis decision making. J Stroke Cerebrovasc Dis 2013;22(4):482–90.
96. Willey JZ, Stillman J, Rivolta JA, et al. Too good to treat? Outcomes in patients not receiving thrombolysis due to mild deficits or rapidly improving symptoms. Int J Stroke 2012;7(3):202–6.
97. Smith EE, Abdullah AR, Petkovska I, et al. Poor outcomes in patients who do not receive intravenous tissue plasminogen activator because of mild or improving ischemic stroke. Stroke 2005;36(11):2497–9.
98. Smith EE, Fonarow GC, Reeves MJ, et al. Outcomes in mild or rapidly improving stroke not treated with intravenous recombinant tissue-type plasminogen activator: findings from Get With The Guidelines-Stroke. Stroke 2011;42(11): 3110–5.
99. Sun MC, Lai TB. Initial stroke severity is the major outcome predictor for patients who do not receive intravenous thrombolysis due to mild or rapidly improving symptoms. ISRN Neurol 2011;2011:947476.
100. Chatzikonstantinou A, Willmann O, Jäger T, et al. Transient ischemic attack patients with fluctuations are at highest risk for early stroke. Cerebrovasc Dis 2009; 27(6):594–8.
101. Ozdemir O, Beletsky V, Chan R, et al. Thrombolysis in patients with marked clinical fluctuations in neurologic status due to cerebral ischemia. Arch Neurol 2008; 65(8):1041–3.
102. Blondin D, Seitz RJ, Rusch O, et al. Clinical impact of MRI perfusion disturbances and normal diffusion in acute stroke patients. Eur J Radiol 2009;71(1):1–10.
103. Greisenegger S, Seyfang L, Austrian Stroke Unit Registry Collaborators, et al. Thrombolysis in patients with mild stroke: results from the Austrian Stroke Unit Registry. Stroke 2014;45(3):765–9.
104. Yeo LL, Ho R, Paliwal P, et al. Intravenously administered tissue plasminogen activator useful in milder strokes? A meta-analysis. J Stroke Cerebrovasc Dis 2014;23(8):2156–62.
105. Amsterdam EA, Wenger NK, Brindis RG, et al. 2014 AHA/ACC guideline for the management of patients with non-ST-elevation acute coronary syndromes: executive summary: a report of the American College of Cardiology/American Heart Association Task Force on practice guidelines. J Am Coll Cardiol 2014; 64(24):2645–87.
106. Antman EM, Anbe DT, Armstrong PW, et al. ACC/AHA guidelines for the management of patients with ST-elevation myocardial infarction—executive summary: a report of the American College of Cardiology/American Heart Association Task Force on Practice Guidelines (writing committee to revise the 1999 guidelines for the management of patients with acute myocardial infarction). Circulation 2004;110(5):588–636.

107. Thornton FJ, Barbul A. Healing in the gastrointestinal tract. Surg Clin North Am 1997;77(3):549–73.
108. Zhang K, Zeng X, Zhu C, et al. Successful thrombolysis in postoperative patients with acute massive pulmonary embolism. Heart Lung Circ 2012;22(2): 100–3.
109. Weiner RA, Daskalakis M, Theodoridou S, et al. Systemic thrombolysis for acute massive pulmonary embolism in the immediate postoperative period after bariatric surgery. Surg Obes Relat Dis 2009;5(2):271–4.
110. Kehl HG, Kececioglu D, Vielhaber H, et al. Left atrial thrombus in a 10-month-old boy—successful thrombolysis with recombinant tissue-type plasminogen activator after open-heart surgery: review of the literature. Intensive Care Med 1996;22(9):968–71.
111. Kawano T, Kajimoto K, Higashi M, et al. Aortic transgraft hemorrhage after intravenous tissue plasminogen activator therapy in patients with acute ischemic stroke. J Stroke Cerebrovasc Dis 2014;23(8):2145–50.
112. Weir CJ, Murray GD, Dyker AG, et al. Is hyperglycaemia an independent predictor of poor outcome after acute stroke? Results of a long-term follow up study. BMJ 1997;314(7090):1303–6.
113. Demchuk AM, Morgenstern LB, Krieger DW, et al. Serum glucose level and diabetes predict tissue plasminogen activator related intracerebral hemorrhage in acute ischemic stroke. Stroke 1999;30(1):34–9.
114. Paciaroni M, Agnelli G, Caso V, et al. Acute hyperglycemia and early hemorrhagic transformation in ischemic stroke. Cerebrovasc Dis 2009;28(2): 119–23.
115. Bruno A, Durkalski VL, Hall CE, et al. The Stroke Hyperglycemia Insulin Network Effort (SHINE) trial protocol: a randomized, blinded, efficacy trial of standard vs. intensive hyperglycemia management in acute stroke. Int J Stroke 2014;9(2): 246–51.
116. Winkler DT, Fluri F, Fuhr P, et al. Thrombolysis in stroke mimics: frequency, clinical characteristics, and outcome. Stroke 2009;40(4):1522–5.
117. Hemmen TM, Meyer BC, McClean TL, et al. Identification of nonischemic stroke mimics among 411 code strokes at the University of California, San Diego, Stroke Center. J Stroke Cerebrovasc Dis 2008;17(1):23–5.
118. Förster A, Griebe M, Wolf ME, et al. How to identify stroke mimics in patients eligible for intravenous thrombolysis? J Neurol 2012;259(7):1347–53.
119. Brunser AM, Illanes S, Lavados PM, et al. Exclusion criteria for intravenous thrombolysis in stroke mimics: an observational study. J Stroke Cerebrovasc Dis 2013;22(7):1140–5.
120. Tsivgoulis G, Alexandrov AV, Chang J, et al. Safety and outcomes of intravenous thrombolysis in stroke mimics: a 6-year, single-care center study and a pooled analysis of reported series. Stroke 2011;42(6):1771–4.
121. Rupprecht S, Schwab M, Fitzek C, et al. Hemispheric hypoperfusion in postictal paresis mimics early brain ischemia. Epilepsy Res 2010;89(2–3):355–9.
122. Sylaja PN, Dzialowski I, Krol A, et al. Role of CT angiography in thrombolysis decision-making for patients with presumed seizure at stroke onset. Stroke 2006;37(3):915–7.
123. Dapprich M, Boessenecker W. Fibrinolysis with alteplase in a pregnant woman with stroke. Cerebrovasc Dis 2002;13(4):290.
124. Wiese KM, Talkad A, Mathews M, et al. Intravenous recombinant tissue plasminogen activator in a pregnant woman with cardioembolic stroke. Stroke 2006; 37(8):2168–9.

125. Mantoan Ritter L, Schuler A, Gangopadhyay R, et al. Successful thrombolysis of stroke with intravenous alteplase in the third trimester of pregnancy. J Neurol 2014;261(3):632–4.
126. Tassi R, Acampa M, Marotta G, et al. Systemic thrombolysis for stroke in pregnancy. Am J Emerg Med 2013;31(2):448.e1–3.
127. Usta IM, Abdallah M, El-Hajj M, et al. Massive subchorionic hematomas following thrombolytic therapy in pregnancy. Obstet Gynecol 2004;103(5 Pt 2):1079–82.
128. Turrentine M, Braems G, Ramirez MM. Use of thrombolytics for the treatment of thromboembolic disease during pregnancy. Obstet Gynecol Surv 1955;50(7): 534–41.
129. Wein TH, Hickenbottom SL, Morgenstern LB, et al. Safety of tissue plasminogen activator for acute stroke in menstruating women. Stroke 2002;33(10):2506–8.
130. Johnston SC, Nguyen-Huynh MN, Schwarz ME, et al. National Stroke Association guidelines for the management of transient ischemic attacks. Ann Neurol 2006;60(3):301–13.

Endovascular Treatment of Acute Ischemic Stroke

Chelsea S. Kidwell, MD[a],*, Reza Jahan, MD[b]

KEYWORDS

- Acute ischemic stroke • Endovascular • MRI • Computed tomography
- Neuroimaging • Penumbra • Thrombolysis

KEY POINTS

- Approaches to endovascular therapy for acute stroke include intra-arterial thrombolytics, bridging intravenous intra-arterial approaches, and mechanical approaches (thrombectomy or aspiration).
- Three randomized trials of endovascular therapy (with first-generation approaches) reported in 2013 did not show a benefit from endovascular treatment compared with standard medical care.
- A single randomized, controlled trial using new-generation stent retriever devices has demonstrated clinical efficacy of endovascular therapy when initiated within 6 hours of onset in patients demonstrating a large vessel occlusion.
- Additional randomized, controlled trials are underway and needed to confirm clinical efficacy with new-generation devices compared with standard care.
- Further properly designed randomized, controlled trials are needed to validate neuroimaging biomarkers to select patients most likely to benefit from treatment.

BACKGROUND

Both animal and human studies have demonstrated that following an occlusion of a cerebral vessel, a region o irreversibly injured core infarct tissue rapidly develops. Surrounding this core is the ischemic penumbra, a region of tissue with diminished blood flow that is still salvageable but at risk of proceeding to infarction if adequate

Dr R. Jahan has the following disclosures: Covidien, Consultant, Member of executive steering committee SWIFT Prime, International Neurointerventional advisor SWIFT Prime, Member of steering committee STARTIS registry; Medina Medical, Chief scientific advisor; Stryker, Speaker's Bureau.

[a] Department of Neurology, University of Arizona, 1501 North Campbell Avenue, Tucson, AZ 85724–5023, USA; [b] Division of Interventional Neuroradiology, Department of Radiology, David Geffen School of Medicine at UCLA, 757 Westwood Plaza, Suite 2129, Los Angeles, CA 90095–7437, USA
* Corresponding author.
E-mail address: ckidwell@email.arizona.edu

Neurol Clin 33 (2015) 401–420
http://dx.doi.org/10.1016/j.ncl.2015.01.005
0733-8619/15/$ – see front matter © 2015 Elsevier Inc. All rights reserved.

neurologic.theclinics.com

blood flow is not quickly restored. Therefore, the goal of recanalization therapies for acute ischemic stroke has been to rapidly remove or disrupt the clot thereby restoring blood flow and salvaging the ischemic penumbra. In 1995, the National Institute of Neurologic Disorders and Stroke (NINDS) trials demonstrated that intravenous thrombolysis with tissue plasminogen activator (IV tPA) improves outcomes in patients treated within 3 hours of symptom onset.[1] Results from the European Cooperative Acute Stroke Study III trial and pooled analysis of IV tPA trials have shown that benefit from treatment with IV tPA may occur up to 4.5 hours from onset.[2,3] However, there are limitations to IV thrombolysis including this relatively narrow time window for treatment, the fact that many patients do not respond to treatment (particularly those with proximal large vessel occlusions), and the approximately 6% risk of symptomatic intracerebral haemorrhage (ICH).

These limitations prompted further interest in developing alternative approaches to vessel recanalization, including endovascular strategies. The first report of endovascular therapy dates back to 1983.[4] Early studies focused on intra-arterial (IA) thrombolysis alone[5] or, following the NINDS IV tPA trial results,[1] combined IA with IV thrombolysis (a bridging approach).[6] However, development of first-generation thrombectomy devices weakened interest in IA thrombolysis because of the potential for rapid recanalization along with hypothetically lower rates of symptomatic hemorrhage with mechanical-based approaches. Unfortunately, the first studies of these first-generation devices were performed as single-arm studies without control arms, and therefore they provided limited data on clinical efficacy and safety compared with untreated patients. Despite this study design, the devices were cleared for removal of cerebral thrombi in patients experiencing acute ischemic stroke by the Food and Drug Administration (FDA) through the Device Branch's 510 k clearance approval process. This in turn led to reimbursement for thrombectomy procedures for acute stroke through Medicare and other insurance providers. Despite the lack of randomized, controlled trials demonstrating either safety or efficacy, use of the devices in clinical practice became widespread. These events made completion of randomized controlled trials difficult, because of lack of equipoise on the provider's end and patient preference to receive an "approved procedure" rather than participate in a research study. An additional critical consequence was that next-generation devices were similarly approved by the same 510 k clearance process without the requirement of randomized controlled trials demonstrating either safety or efficacy.

However, in 2013, three randomized, controlled trials of endovascular therapy using first-generation devices were reported.[7–9] Although all three had different designs and time windows, none of the three trials demonstrated efficacy of endovascular procedures compared with the control arms. Despite the recognized limitations of these trials, the results substantially increased doubt concerning the routine use of these procedures in clinical practice, leading to a greater recognized need for further randomized trials with new-generation devices and return to equipoise regarding their efficacy. In late 2014, the first randomized controlled trial using new-generation stent retrievers was reported demonstrating improved functional outcome in the endovascular arm. Results of additional randomized trials using new-generation devices are pending at the time of this publication.

SUMMARY OF ENDOVASCULAR TRIALS FOR ACUTE ISCHEMIC STROKE

Although a large number of case series have been reported in the literature, this section focuses on the main pivotal, multicenter, prospective studies of endovascular therapies to date for acute ischemic stroke. **Table 1** provides a summary of study designs, patient characteristics, and outcome measures (with outcome measures harmonized to the extent possible to allow comparison across studies).

Chemical Thrombolysis (Intra-arterial Thrombolysis)

Prolyse in Acute Cerebral Thromboembolism II (PROACT II) was a phase III, randomized, controlled, open-label, blinded outcome trial of IA recombinant prourokinase plus IV heparin versus IV heparin alone plus angiography initiated within 6 hours of symptom onset.[10] Only patients with angiographically proved middle cerebral artery occlusions were enrolled. In the primary intention-to-treat analysis, 40% of patients treated with IA prourokinase had a good outcome (Day 90 modified Rankin scale [mRS] score, 0–2) compared with 25% of the control arm ($P = .04$). Recanalization as measured by a Thrombolysis in Myocardial Infarction (TIMI) score of 2 to 3 was achieved in 66% of patients in the IA arm. Mortality rates were similar between groups (25% prourokinase arm vs 27% control arm). However, symptomatic hemorrhage tended to be higher in the prourokinase arm at 10% compared with 2% in control subjects ($P = .06$). Because the FDA requires two confirmatory trials for drug approval and the sponsor chose not to pursue an additional trial, IA prourokinase was not approved by the FDA for treatment of acute ischemic stroke. Currently, alternative thrombolytics are used for IA therapy with the most common being tPA.

A second, randomized, controlled trial of IA thrombolysis was conducted in Japan and reported in 2007 after early termination of the trial because of approval of IV tPA by Japanese regulatory agencies. The Middle Cerebral Artery Embolism Local Fibrinolytic Intervention Trial randomized 114 patients (original target sample size was 200) with M1 or M2 middle cerebral artery occlusions demonstrated on angiography to urokinase or best medical management.[11] Although urokinase patients tended to have more frequent good outcomes at 90 days (mRS, 0–2), this did not reach statistical significance (49% vs 39%; $P = .35$). Partial or complete recanalization was achieved in 74% of the urokinase-treated patients. Notably, mortality in both groups was substantially lower than in all other endovascular trials to date (urokinase arm, 5.3%; control arm, 3.5%). Symptomatic hemorrhage rates, however, were comparable with other trials (9% prourokinase arm, 2% control arm; $P = .21$).

Mechanical Approaches

First-generation thrombectomy devices

The first thrombectomy device developed specifically for acute ischemic stroke was the Merci retriever (Concentric Medical, Fremont, CA).[12] The first-generation devices were designed like a corkscrew and were evaluated in single-arm studies (**Fig. 1**). The results of the first Mechanical Embolus Removal in Cerebral Ischemia (MERCI) trials were reported as a single study, although they were conducted in two parts, with part II having expanded eligibility criteria and longer follow-up.[13] A total of 151 patients were enrolled within 8 hours of onset with a proximal intracranial large vessel occlusion (including posterior circulation). Ten patients did not undergo the thrombectomy procedure. TIMI 2 to 3 recanalization was achieved in 48% of patients treated with the retriever alone and in 60% when adjunctive therapy was included. Good functional outcome (90-day mRS) was reported in 28% of patients overall with significantly higher rates in those with recanalization versus those without (46% vs 10%; $P = .0001$). Symptomatic hemorrhage occurred in 8% of patients and 90-day mortality was high at 43.5%.

The subsequent Multi-MERCI trial was also a single-arm, multicenter study of thrombectomy within 8 hours of onset in patients with a large vessel occlusion.[14] Multi-MERCI differed in several ways from MERCI: patients treated with IV tPA with

Table 1
Pivotal acute ischemic stroke endovascular clinical studies and trials

	Study	Design	TW (h)	TTT (h)	N	Treatments	Median NIHSS	Day 90 mRS 0–2 (%)	Day 90 Mortality (%)	sICH (%)	Recanalization
IA thrombolytics	PROACT II	Randomized, controlled	6	4.5	180	IA prourokinase vs IV heparin + angiography	17	40 / 25	25 / 27	10 / 2	66% (TIMI 2–3) / 18%
	MELT	Randomized, controlled	6	3.8	114[a]	IA urokinase vs control	14	49 / 39	5 / 3.5	9 / 2	74% / NA
First-generation mechanical devices	MERCI	Single arm	8	4.3	151 (ITT) 141 (PP)	First-generation Merci Retriever (X5, X6)	20 (mean)	28	43.5	8	48%/60%[b]
	Multi-MERCI	Single arm	8	4.3	164	First- and second-generation Merci Retriever	19	36	34	10	55%/68%[b]
Bridging approaches	IMS	Single arm (vs NINDS trial arms)	3	2.3 (IV) 3.5 (IA)	80	0.6 mg/kg IV tPA + up to 22 mg IA tPA	18	43	16	6.3	56% (TICI2–3)
	IMS II	Single arm (vs NINDS trial arms)	3	2.4 (IV) NR (IA)	81	0.6 mg/kg IV tPA + up to 22 mg IA tPA	19	46	16	9.9	60% (TICI 2–3)
	IMS III	Randomized, controlled	3	2.0 (IV) 3.5 (IA)	656	IV tPA vs IV tPA + endovascular	16.5	38.7 / 40.8	21.6 / 19.1	5.9 / 6.2	(TICI 2–3) 65% internal carotid artery 81% M1 70% M2 77% multiple M2

Stent retrievers	SWIFT	Randomized, parallel group	8	4.9 SR / 5.3 MR	113[c]	Solitaire vs Merci Retriever	18	37 / 28	18 / 44	2 / 11	69% (TIMI 2–3) / 30%
	TREVO	Open-label, randomized, controlled	8	4.4 (IA)	178	Trevo vs Merci Retriever	19	40 / 22	33 / 24	7 / 9	86% (TICI 2a–3) / 60%
	MR CLEAN	Multicenter, randomized, controlled	6	1.4 (IV) / 4.3 (IA)	500	Endovascular + usual vs usual	17–18	32.6 vs 19.1	21 / 22	7.7 / 6.4	58.7 (TICI 2b–3) / 80.6 (TICI 2a–3)
Aspiration devices	Penumbra	Single arm	8	4.3	125	Penumbra System	18 (mean)	25	33	11	82% (TIMI 2–3)
IV vs IA approaches	SYNTHESIS	Randomized, blinded outcome	4.5	2.75 (IV) / 3.75 (IA)	362	IV tPA vs any endovascular[d]	13	46[e] / 42	10 / 14	6 / 6	Not reported
Imaging-based trials	DEFUSE 2	Single arm, cohort	12	6.2 (TM) / 4.7 (no TM)	138[f]	Any endovascular[f]	16	40	18	10	77% (TICI 2a–3)
	MR RESCUE	Randomized, controlled, blinded outcome	8	2.2 (IV)[g] / 6.4 (IA)	118	Standard medical care vs endovascular[g]	17	20 / 19	24 / 19	4 / 5	NA / 69% (TICI 2a–3)

Abbreviations: IMS, Interventional Management of Stroke; ITT, intention to treat; MELT, Middle Cerebral Artery Embolism Local Fibrinolytic Intervention; MERCI, Mechanical Embolus Removal in Cerebral Ischemia; MR, Merci Retriever; MR CLEAN, Multicenter Randomized Clinical Trial of Endovascular Treatment for Acute Ischemic Stroke in the Netherlands; MR RESCUE, Mechanical Retrieval and Recanalization of Stroke Clots Using Embolectomy; mRS, modified Rankin scale; NIHSS, National Institutes of Health Stroke Scale; PP, per protocol analysis; PROACT, Prolyse in Acute Cerebral Thromboembolism; sICH, symptomatic intracerebral hemorrhage; SR, Solitaire Retriever; SWIFT, Solitaire With the Intention For Thrombectomy; TM, target mismatch; TTT, time to treatment (start; for endovascular therapy, time to groin puncture is most commonly reported measure); TREVO, Thrombectomy Revascularization of Large Vessel Occlusions in Acute Ischemic Stroke; TW, time window.

a Stopped early with approval of IV tPA in Japan.
b Second rate included use of adjunctive IA thrombolytics.
c Stopped prematurely after reaching efficacy stopping rule.
d Any endovascular included mechanical clot disruption or retrieval, IA tPA, or a combination (only 14% treated with stent retrievers); initiation within 6 hours.
e Primary outcome measure was mRS 0–1, which did not differ between groups.
f Only 98 of 138 underwent endovascular treatment; endovascular treatment included Merci device, Penumbra system, and IA thrombolysis; patients treated with IV tPA were eligible.
g IV tPA failures allows in arms; TTT for IV is only those cases treated with IV tPA and time to IA is only for the embolectomy arm; endovascular arm included first-generation devices but not stent retrievers; randomization.

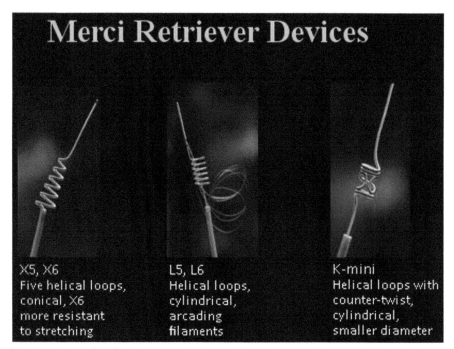

Fig. 1. Images of different generations of the Merci Retriever. (*Courtesy of* Stryker, Kalamazoo, MI; with permission.)

a persistent occlusion were eligible for enrollment and most patients were treated with the next-generation L5 Retriever, which included monofilaments that attached proximally and distally to the helical nitinol coils (see **Fig. 1**). Of the 161 subjects enrolled, 36% had good outcome at 90 days (mRS, 0–2). Day 90 mortality was still high at 34% but lower than that reported in the first MERCI study, and symptomatic hemorrhage rate was 10%. Overall recanalization rates were also higher than in the first study at 55% for the device alone, and 68% after adjunctive IA therapy.

Bridging approaches

An innovative bridging (IV to IA) approach to acute stroke therapy was first tested in the Emergency Management of Stroke (EMS) bridging trial.[6] This approach combined early treatment with lower dose IV tPA (0.6 mg/kg) followed by IA delivery of the thrombolytic at the site of the clot. The EMS study of 35 patients demonstrated greater rates of complete recanalization in patients treated with the bridging approach compared with IA tPA alone (6 of 11 vs 1 of 10) in patients treated within 3 hours of symptom onset. The EMS study was followed by the first Interventional Management of Stroke (IMS) study.[15] A total of 80 patients with National Institutes of Health Stroke Scale (NIHSS) scores greater than 10 were treated with bridging therapy (two-third dose IV tPA followed by IA tPA up to 22 mg), again with treatment initiated within 3 hours of onset. Outcomes were compared with historical controls (placebo and IV tPA arms from the NINDS tPA trials).[1] Good outcomes, including mRS 0 to 1 and 0 to 2, were higher in the IMS cohort compared with the NINDS placebo-treated subjects (30% vs 18%, and 43% vs 28%, respectively), but were similar to the IV tPA group. Symptomatic hemorrhage rate was 6.3%, again similar to the NINDS IV tPA rate.

Mortality tended to be lower in the IMS group (16%) compared with both arms of the NINDS trial (24% placebo; 21% tPA). Median time to IV tPA treatment was 140 minutes and to IA tPA was 212 minutes.

The feasibility and safety of the bridging approach was further evaluated in the IMS II study.[16] Study design was similar to the first IMS trial except that IA tPA infusion could be delivered with the EKOS (EKOS Corporation, Bothell, WA) small vessel ultrasound microinfusion system or a standard microcatheter. Of the 81 subjects enrolled, median NIHSS score was 19. Results were remarkably similar to those from IMS: median time to IV tPA start was 142 minutes, 3-month mortality rate was 16%, and good outcomes were better than NINDS placebo group. Good outcomes were also better than the NINDS IV tPA group as measured by the Barthel Index and Global Test statistical. Symptomatic hemorrhage was slightly higher than IMS at 9.9%. Overall recanalization rate was 60% as measured by a Thrombolysis in Cerebral Infarction (TICI) score of 2 to 3. Compared with patients in IMS treated with a standard microcatheter, use of the EKOS system did not significantly accelerate or improve overall recanalization rates.

The IMS III trial was designed to be a definitive phase III randomized, controlled trial of bridging therapy compared with standard IV tPA within 3 hours of symptom onset.[7] Endovascular therapy could consist of IA tPA or clot retrieval with the Merci Retriever. Late in the trial, additional devices were allowed including the Penumbra System (Penumbra, Inc, Alameda, CA) and stent retrievers. The investigators planned to enroll a total of 900 subjects in a 2:1 ratio to bridging therapy or IV tPA alone, with the primary outcome measure being good outcome at 90 days (mRS, 0–2). Following an interim analysis, the study was stopped early because of futility after 656 subjects were enrolled. Overall good outcome was similar in both groups: 40.8% of patients in the endovascular arm compared with 38.7% with IV tPA alone. There were no significant differences in the prespecified subgroup of patients with NIHSS scores of 20 or greater or those less than 20. Day-90 mortality was similar in both groups (endovascular, 19.1%; IV tPA, 21.6), as were symptomatic hemorrhage rates (6.2% vs 5.9%, respectively). Because stent retrievers were only available and allowed in the latter portion of the trial, they were used in only 5 of 334 patients that underwent interventions.

An important finding demonstrated in the IMS trials was the association between time to reperfusion and good outcome. In an analysis from IMS I and II, for cases with reperfusion of the middle cerebral artery or distal internal carotid artery, the probability of good clinical outcome decreased as time to angiographic reperfusion increased; within 7 hours the probability approached that of cases without reperfusion.[17] In a similar analysis of cases from IMS III, increased time to reperfusion was again associated with decreased likelihood of good outcome with the adjusted relative risk of 0.88 for every 30-minute delay.[18] In IMS III, greater recanalization rates were demonstrated in the endovascular arm compared with IV tPA; however, this did not result in better outcomes.

Aspiration thrombectomy devices

The Penumbra System (**Fig. 2**) was developed as an alternative mechanical approach to thrombectomy. The system allows for thrombus debulking and aspiration and direct thrombus extraction. The Penumbra Pivotal Stroke Trial, reported in 2009, enrolled 125 patients within 8 hours of symptom onset.[19] Both anterior and posterior (vertebrobasilar) circulation occlusions were eligible as were IV tPA failures. Mean NIHSS score was 17.6. A postprocedural TIMI 2 to 3 score was achieved in 82% of patients. Good outcome (mRS, 0–2) was reported in 25%, Day-90 mortality was 33%, and

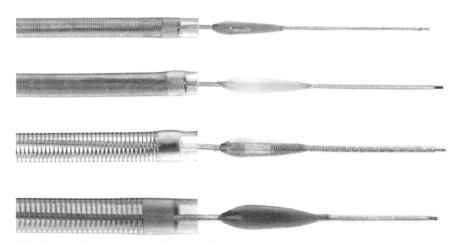

Fig. 2. Images demonstrating the Penumbra System. (*Courtesy of* Penumbra, Inc, Alameda, CA; with permission.)

symptomatic ICH occurred in 11% of subjects. Of note, baseline ASPECTS score correlated strongly with outcome in this study.[20]

Stent retrievers

In 2012, the results of two trials of new-generation stent retrievers were reported. Stent retrievers (**Fig. 3**) were developed as self-expanding stents designed to entrap the clot when deployed within the occluded vessel. Both trials randomized patients to new-generation devices or to the Merci retrievers and therefore no conclusions could be drawn regarding efficacy of the procedure versus standard care. In the Solitaire With the Intention For Thrombectomy (SWIFT) trial, 113 patients with a median NIHSS score of 18 were randomized within 8 hours to treatment with the Solitaire stent retriever (Covidien Neurovascular, Irvine, CA) or the Merci Retrieval System.[21] The trial was stopped early after reaching its efficacy stopping rule. The primary outcome, TIMI 2 to 3 flow in all treatable vessels without symptomatic ICH, was achieved in 61% of the Solitaire group compared with 24% in the Merci group. In addition, good clinical outcome (combined measure of mRS 0–2, or equal to the prestroke mRS if the pre-stroke mRS was >2, or NIHSS score improvement of 10 points or more) was greater

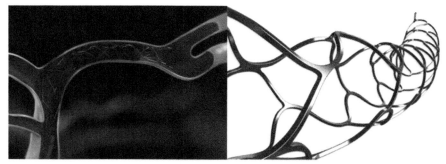

Fig. 3. Images of the Solitaire stent retriever (*left image*) and Trevo ProVue Retriever (*right image*). (*Courtesy of* [*left image*] Covidien Neurovascular, Irvine, CA; and [*right image*] Stryker, Kalamazoo, MI; with permission.)

in the Solitaire group (58% vs 33%). Day-90 mortality was lower (17% vs 38%), and symptomatic ICH rates tended to be lower (11% vs 2%) in the Solitaire group.

In the second trial, Thrombectomy Revascularization of Large Vessel Occlusions in Acute Ischemic Stroke (TREVO) II, 178 patients with a median NIHSS score of 19 were randomized to treatment with the Trevo Retriever (Stryker Neurovascular, Kalamazoo, MI) or the Merci Retriever within 8 hours of symptom onset.[22] The primary endpoint of TICI 2 to 3 revascularization was achieved in 86% of the Trevo group compared with 60% of the Merci group. Good outcome (Day-90 mRS) occurred in 40% of the Trevo group compared with 22% of the Merci group. Symptomatic ICH and mortality did not differ significantly between the groups. In combination, the TREVO and SWIFT trials demonstrate superior efficacy and safety of the new-generation devices compared with the Merci Retriever; however, without standard care controls arms, no conclusions could be drawn regarding overall device efficacy compared with standard medical care.

Most recently, results of a new randomized, controlled trial, the Multicenter Randomized Clinical trial of Endovascular Treatment for Acute Ischemic Stroke in the Netherlands (MR CLEAN), have been published.[23] In this trial, 16 centers randomized 500 patients with anterior circulation ischemic strokes to endovascular therapy plus standard care or standard care alone. Inclusion required evidence of a large vessel occlusion on pretreatment vessel imaging and ability to initiate endovascular therapy within 6 hours of symptom onset. Usual care included treatment with IV tPA within 4.5 hours of onset, which was administered in 89% of patients across both arms. The primary outcome analysis demonstrated that endovascular therapy was associated with a shift to improved function at 90 days as assessed by the mRS with an adjusted odds ratio of 1.67 (95% confidence interval, 1.21–2.30). As a secondary analysis, good functional outcome, defined as a dichotomized mRS 0 to 2, was achieved in 32.6% of patients in the endovascular arm compared with 19.1% in the usual care arm. Median time to groin puncture was 260 minutes in the endovascular arm, and therapy involved retrievable stents in 81.5% of cases. Revascularization, defined as TICI 2b to 3, was achieved in 58.7% of interventional cases. There was no difference in overall mortality or rate of symptomatic hemorrhage between groups; however, there was a higher rate of new stroke in a different territory in the intervention arm (5.6% vs 0.4%). On 24-hour vessel imaging, there was no evidence of occlusion in 75.4% of patients in the intervention arm compared with 32.9% of patients in the control arm. In patients with Day 5 to 7 computed tomography imaging available, final infarct volume was smaller in the endovascular compared with the standard care arm (49 vs 79 mL).

Intravenous versus intra-arterial approaches

The SYNTHESIS (Intra-arterial Versus Systemic Thrombolysis for Acute Ischemic Stroke) Expansion trial was one of the three neutral randomized, controlled trials of endovascular therapy for acute ischemic stroke reported in 2013. SYNTHESIS randomized 362 patients within 4.5 hours of onset to endovascular therapy or IV tPA. Endovascular therapy included IA thrombolysis, mechanical approaches, or a combination at the discretion of the treating physician. Overall, there was no difference between groups in the primary outcome measure of Day-90 survival free of disability (mRS, 0–1; 30.4% for endovascular versus 34.8% for IV tPA; $P = .016$). Similarly, symptomatic hemorrhage rates were the same between both groups at 6% as was mortality (10% IV tPA vs 14% endovascular). Recanalization rates in the endovascular arm were not reported. Of note, 16 patients in the endovascular arm did not receive treatment, and the most patients in the endovascular arm were treated with either IA tPA, mechanical clot disruption, or first-generation devices.

Imaging-Based Approaches

Two trials exploring the role of imaging-based selection for endovascular therapy have been reported to date. DEFUSE (Diffusion and Perfusion Imaging Evaluation for Understanding Stroke Evolution) 2 was a prospective cohort study of patients receiving endovascular therapy for acute ischemic stroke within 12 hours of symptom onset. All patients underwent a pretreatment MRI that was processed at the site using an automated analysis program to establish whether or not they had a target mismatch profile suggesting salvageable tissue. Follow-up MRIs were performed within 12 hours of the procedure to determine if reperfusion had occurred. Of the 138 subjects enrolled, median NIHSS score was 16, a total of 98 underwent endovascular treatment, and 99 could be assessed for reperfusion. Overall, 40% of patients had a good outcome (mRS, 0–2), 10% had symptomatic hemorrhages, and mortality rate was 18%. A TICI 2a to 3 recanalization rate was achieved in 77% of subjects. The investigators reported that patients with target mismatch had a greater likelihood of favorable clinical response, which was associated with reperfusion. However, numbers of patients in some of the groups were very small and importantly, without a control arm, no firm conclusions could be drawn regarding treatment efficacy.

MR RESCUE (Mechanical Retrieval and Recanalization of Stroke Clots Using Embolectomy) was a third randomized, controlled trial reported in 2013. The goals of MR RESCUE were to test the penumbral imaging selection hypothesis and to demonstrate efficacy of thrombectomy for acute ischemic stroke compared with standard care. A total of 118 patients were randomized to embolectomy versus standard care with randomization stratified by favorable penumbral imaging pattern (substantial salvageable tissue and small infarct core) on nonpenumbral pattern. Penumbral pattern was determined in real time at the site using an automated image analysis program using multivariate voxel-based models of tissue outcome rather than the mismatch model.[24] The mean time to enrollment was 5.5 hours and median NIHSS was 17. Using a shift analysis, the mean 90-day mRS (primary outcome measure) did not differ across groups. Overall mortality was 21% and rate of symptomatic ICH 4%, neither of which differed across groups. In the embolectomy group, TICI 2a to 3 recanalization rate was 69%. The investigators concluded that a favorable penumbral pattern did not identify patients who would benefit from endovascular therapy and that endovascular therapy in the trial was not superior to standard medical care in patients treated with first-generation devices within an 8-hour time window. As with the other randomized trials to date, the trial tested mainly first-generation devices. Additional limitations included the long time frame required for study recruitment, the relatively late time to endovascular treatment from symptom onset (mean time to groin puncture, 6.2 hours), and the relatively large predicted infarct core even within the penumbral group (median predicted core volume, 60.2 mL for entire cohort, 36.6 mL for penumbral group, and 117.5 mL for nonpenumbral group).

However, several notable observations were made in MR RESCUE. Patients with favorable penumbral patterns had significantly better outcomes than those patients with nonpenumbral patterns regardless of treatment. Second, among patients with follow-up imaging at Day 7, there were better outcomes in patients with imaging evidence of revascularization/reperfusion regardless of treatment group. Without the control arm, it would not have been evident that the benefit of revascularization was not a direct treatment effect. The investigators postulated that patients with a penumbral pattern at late time windows have sufficient collaterals to sustain the penumbra until eventual spontaneous recanalization occurs, and therefore it is possible that revascularization therapies may not be beneficial in this group at this late window. Finally, MR RESCUE demonstrated that there was no evidence of harm in the nonpenumbral patients who randomized to endovascular therapy. This is important for design of future trials testing the penumbral selection hypothesis (ie, the argument that it is unethical to treat nonpenumbral pattern patients because of increased risk of poor outcomes has been disproven).

AREAS OF CONTROVERSY, COUNTERARGUMENTS

The history of endovascular treatment of acute ischemic stroke emphasizes important concepts regarding clinical trial design, evidence-based medicine, scientific equipoise, and the regulatory approval process. The failure to include standard care control arms in clinical trials, in conjunction with the FDA Device Branch's 510 k clearance process, engendered and promoted a perception of device efficacy despite lack of evidence. This lack of equipoise was compounded by subsequent Medicare reimbursement for the procedure. Clinicians and investigators not only had a financial incentive to perform procedures (rather than participate in randomized controlled trials), but also raised ethical questions with regard to performing randomized, controlled trials that included a standard medical care arm with a concern for harm in this group.

The neutral results in 2013 of the three randomized trials with standard medical care arms highlighted the paucity of data demonstrating improved outcomes for endovascular therapy compared with standard medical care, despite widespread use of these procedures in clinical practice.[7-9] All three of the trials were criticized for being outdated by the time of publication because they were largely based on first-generation devices. This was because of rapid changes in technology in the face of slow recruitment in randomized trials, and the lengthy regulatory process required to introduce new devices into clinical trials. On the heels of these trials, there was a generalized recognition of a need for greater equipoise and a renewed interest in randomized, controlled trials of the new-generation devices.[25]

These negative randomized trials also raised important questions regarding the FDA Device Branch's 510 k clearance process and reimbursement for procedures by Medicare and other insurance providers. It was suggested that a moratorium be placed on reimbursement for endovascular procedures outside of randomized clinical trials.[25] This would have markedly facilitated recruitment in the IMS III and MR RESCUE and would have likely mitigated concerns regarding selection bias.

In contrast, MR CLEAN was completed in 3 years and 4 months during which there was widespread availability of new-generation devices at participating centers. Furthermore, all centers providing endovascular therapy for stroke in the Netherlands participated in the trial. Most notably, in the latter portion of the trial, reimbursement by insurance companies required participation in the trial.

The positive results of MR CLEAN compared with prior trials are likely multifactorial. Although the trial largely used new-generation devices, the rate of revascularization was modest compared with other series but was higher than that reported in IMS III.[7,21,22] In contrast to IMS III, MR CLEAN required evidence of a large vessel occlusion before randomization, and time from tPA administration to randomization was longer than allowed in IMS III. As such, it is possible IMS III included more patients who may not have benefited from endovascular therapy compared with MR CLEAN (ie, tPA responders or patients without a large vessel occlusion). Several aspects of the patient cohort in MR CLEAN are noteworthy: baseline systolic blood pressure was relatively low (145–146 mm Hg), time to IV tPA treatment substantially shorter than most prior trials (85–87 minutes), and baseline ASPECTS score relatively high (median, 9). It is unclear if any of these characteristics impacted results. Completion of further randomized, controlled trials is still needed to confirm the positive results of MR CLEAN and their generalizability to different populations and health care systems.

The role of advanced imaging for selection of patients for endovascular therapies remains highly controversial. IMS III and SYNTHESIS were criticized for enrolling patients without the requirement of vessel imaging to demonstrate a target occlusion.[7,26] It has been argued that without this requirement, the patient pool was diluted with patients who could still benefit from IV tPA but not endovascular therapy, thereby limiting power to show a treatment benefit. The positive results of MR CLEAN further support the role of vessel imaging as a selection criterion for endovascular therapy.

The role of penumbral imaging for selection of patients for acute stroke therapies remains controversial.[27] Early animal studies demonstrating the presence of an ischemic penumbra for several hours or more following an acute stroke led to the notion that advanced imaging could be used to identify patients likely to benefit from recanalization therapies, irrespective of time windows. With the introduction of diffusion-perfusion MRI and subsequently perfusion computed tomography into clinical practice, simplistic, operational approaches to defining the penumbra were proposed and adopted in clinical trials without rigorous studies confirming their validity.[28]

Interpretation of the contrasting results from DEFUSE 2 and MR RESCUE remains a controversial topic.[8,29] The DEFUSE 2 investigators concluded that patients with target mismatch had a greater likelihood of favorable clinical response, which was associated with reperfusion, a finding that was not replicated in MR RESCUE. MR RESCUE used multivariate voxel-based models for predicting infarct core and penumbral pattern. The predicted core in the penumbral group of patients in MR RESCUE was substantially greater than that in DEFUSE 2. In both trials there was concern for selection bias. In the case of MR RESCUE, patients less likely to benefit from therapy may have been enrolled, whereas in DEFUSE 2, patients more likely to benefit from therapy may have been selected. The small number of patients in DEFUSE 2, especially in the subgroup analyses, also raises concern, particularly when there is no control arm. It is also possible that the low rates of TICI 2b–3 recanalization in MR RESCUE obscured the ability to show a treatment benefit in penumbral patients. Alternatively, it is possible that the penumbral imaging hypothesis for patient selection for late revascularization for ischemic stroke is flawed. In later time windows, a favorable penumbral pattern may be a biomarker for a good outcome because of the presence of more vigorous collateral vessels and therefore greater tolerance of occlusion, increased likelihood of eventual spontaneous recanalization, and good final outcome.[8]

More recently, imaging proponents have focused attention on the volume of core, irreversibly injured tissue, and the presence of a target vessel occlusion as the most important imaging selection biomarkers for acute stroke revascularization therapies. Although use of the selection biomarkers as inclusion criteria has the advantage of increasing the likelihood of a positive trial by enriching the patient population with subjects most likely to benefit, there is the risk that excluded patients may also have benefited if the correct biomarker was not chosen or optimized.

It should also be noted that most trials to date have either included very few patients with vertebrobasilar occlusions or have excluded these patients altogether. Outcomes in patients with posterior circulation occlusions, particularly those in the basilar artery, tend to be far worse. Some investigators have also postulated that the pathophysiology of penumbra and collaterals may differ from the anterior circulation, and therefore the time window for treatment may also differ. As such, it can be argued that separate trials should be conducted to test endovascular therapy in the posterior circulation. A prospective registry conducted from 2002 to 2007 did not support superiority of endovascular approaches over IV tPA in patients with basilar occlusions.[30] The Basilar Artery International Cooperation Study is an ongoing randomized controlled open-label phase III trial that will examine the efficacy and safety of endovascular therapy in patients treated with IV tPA.

Finally, lack of standardization of outcome measures has also hampered interpretation and comparison of results across clinical trials. Although mRS is the most widely used measure to assess outcomes, it is frequently analyzed with different cutpoints or using a shift analysis approach. In the SWIFT trial, the investigators used novel approaches to define outcomes.[21] The primary outcome measure was successful recanalization with no symptomatic hemorrhage. Good neurologic outcome was defined as mRS of 2 or less, or equal to the prestroke mRS if the prestroke mRS was greater than 2, or NIHSS score improvement of 10 points or more. Good outcome using this novel definition was achieved in 58% of patients treated with the Solitaire device, compared with a rate of 37% using the traditional cutpoint of mRS 0 to 2. Approaches to measuring revascularization have also varied widely. Adoption of the TIMI scale for the cerebral vasculature proved problematic and new scales, most notably the TICI, have been used in most recent trials. However, variations on the scale, lack of blinded core laboratory assessments, and differing opinions on the most meaningful cutpoints continue to hamper adoption of standard approaches.

CONCLUSIONS AND LEVELS OF EFFICACY

Endovascular therapy with new-generation stent retriever devices for treatment of acute stroke remains promising, particularly in light of a recent positive randomized, controlled trial using new-generation stent retrievers demonstrating improved clinical outcomes compared with standard medical care. Although further trials are needed, based on this trial, there is category T2 evidence that endovascular therapy with stent retrievers plus usual care is beneficial when initiated within 6 hours of onset in patients with a demonstrable large vessel anterior circulation occlusion. Furthermore, there is category T1 evidence demonstrating that the stent retrievers have clinical efficacy compared with the Merci Retriever. For first-generation devices, there is category T1 evidence from randomized, controlled trials that these procedures are ineffective compared with current standard medical care including IV tPA alone for eligible patients. The role of advanced, multimodal imaging including penumbral imaging for selecting candidates for treatment of endovascular therapies remains unknown and unproved. The results of further endovascular trials using new-generation stent retrievers are highly anticipated (**Table 2**). Some of these new trials are designed to demonstrate clinical efficacy compared with standard care; however, others are prone to the same pitfalls of prior studies including lack of standard care control arms and use of nonvalidated imaging selection biomarkers as inclusion criteria.

PROCEDURES

For endovascular therapies for acute ischemic stroke, there is substantial technical variation among different practitioners with no definite scientific evidence to justify a particular approach.

Table 2
Current or planned multicenter endovascular trials for acute stroke (registries not included)

Trial Name	Design	Sample Size	Treatment Arms	Time Window	Primary Outcome	Locations (Sponsor)
BASICS	Multicenter, randomized, controlled	750	IV tPA + ET vs IV tPA for basilar occlusion	4.5 h	Day 90 mRS	Europe (BASICS Study Group)
DAWN	Multicenter, randomized, controlled[a]	500	Medical management vs Trevo Stent Retriever	6–24 h	Day 90 mRS	United States (Stryker Neurovascular)
ESCAPE	Multicenter, randomized, controlled[a]	500	Endovascular therapy ± IV tPA vs medical management	12 h	Day 90 mRS 0–2 or NIHSS 0–2	Canada, United States, Europe, Asia (University of Calgary)
EXTEND-IA	Multicenter, randomized, controlled, radiologically selected[a]	150	Solitaire Retriever + IV tPA vs IV tPA	6 h	Reperfusion at 72 h without sICH	Australia, New Zealand (National Stroke Research Institute)
PISTE	Multicenter, randomized, controlled	800	IV tPA + ET vs IV tPA	4.5 h	Day 90 mRS	Britain (NHS Greater Glasgow and Clyde)
REVASCAT	Multicenter, randomized, controlled	690	Solitaire Retriever + IV tPA vs medical management	8 h	Day 90 mRS (Shift)	Spain (Covidien)
SWIFT Prime	Multicenter, randomized, controlled	833	Solitaire Retriever + IV tPA vs IV tPA	6 h	Day 90 mRS	United States, Europe (Covidien)
THERAPY	Multicenter, randomized, controlled	692	Penumbra System + IV tPA vs IV tPA	4.5 h	Day 90 mRS	United States (Penumbra Inc)
THRACE	Multicenter, randomized, controlled	480	IV tPA + ET vs IV tPA	4 h	Day 90 mRS	France (Central Hospital, Nancy, France)
THRILL	Multicenter, randomized, controlled	600	Stent retrievers vs medical management	8 h	Day 90 mRS (Shift)	Austria, Germany (Covidien, Stryker)

Abbreviations: BASICS, Basilar Artery International Cooperation Study; DAWN, Trevo and Medical Management versus Medical Management Alone in Wake Up and Late Presenting Strokes; ESCAPE, Endovascular Treatment for Small Core and Proximal Occlusion Ischemic Stroke; ET, endovascular therapy; EXTEND-IA, Extending the Time for Thrombolysis in Emergency Neurologic Deficits - Intra-Arterial; PISTE, Pragmatic Ischaemic Stroke Thrombectomy Evaluation; REVASCAT, Endovascular Revascularization With Solitaire Device versus Best Medical Therapy in Anterior Circulation Stroke Within 8 Hours; sICH, symptomatic intracerebral hemorrhage; SWIFT Prime, Solitaire FR as Primary Treatment for Acute Ischemic Stroke; THERAPY, Assess the Penumbra System in the Treatment of Acute Stroke; THRACE, Trial and Cost Effectiveness Evaluation of Intra-arterial Thrombectomy in Acute Ischemic Stroke; THRILL, Thrombectomy in stroke patients ineligible for IV tPA.

[a] Imaging-based inclusion criteria.

General Considerations

Systemic anticoagulation

Systemic anticoagulation with heparin is routinely used in all cerebrovascular interventional procedures; however, in the setting of acute ischemic stroke, with few exceptions, most recent trials have not required systemic anticoagulation.[8,21,22] The use of systemic anticoagulation has often been left at the discretion of the treating physician and per standard institutional practice. Although the rationale for administration of heparin has been to prevent thromboembolic events related to placement of catheters in the cerebral vasculature, this is balanced by the risk of concern for hemorrhage, particularly in patients who have received system IV tPA. In addition, in the setting of ischemic stroke, it has been hypothesized that the anticoagulation during the procedure will prevent further thrombus formation in the already occluded vessel. In fact, the PROACT study showed that heparin augmented the thrombolytic effect of Pro-Urokinase in achieving thrombolysis.[31] Recommendations for anticoagulation vary, but most tend to follow the PROACT II protocol with a heparin bolus of 2000 IU followed by 500 IU per hour thereafter.[10] In IMS III, the bolus dose was also 2000 IU but the maintenance dose was 450 IU per hour.[7] The rates of symptomatic hemorrhage in these two studies seem to indicate that either approach is an acceptable protocol. The infusion is discontinued at the end of the procedure.

Heparin flush solutions for angiography and intervention

Heparinized saline solutions are routinely used for continuous flushing of catheters during angiography and cerebral interventional procedures. These should not contain glucose. In the PROACT II and IMS III trials, heparin flush solutions contained 1 U/mL heparin in 0.9% sodium chloride and were infused at 60 and 30 mL/h, respectively.[7,10] Antithrombotic agents were otherwise prohibited for the first 24 hours.

Preintervention diagnostic catheter angiogram

Many centers now routinely perform noninvasive vessel imaging at the time that parenchymal imaging is obtained, obviating detailed cerebral angiograms. Nevertheless, there are still circumstances where complete cerebral angiography is necessary in this setting. The goals of cerebral angiography are to identify the site and extent of occlusion, identify collaterals through the circle of Willis, identify leptomeningeal collaterals to the affected territory, and assess brachiocephalic vessels for access to the occluded vessel.

Typically the occluded territory is the last vessel studied so as to have a complete picture of the collateral flow. In addition, the angiogram provides important information in planning the strategy for intervention and determining the risks of the procedure, in particular the technical risks in cases with tortuous anatomy.

General anesthesia versus local anesthesia

Recently, several studies have suggested the choice of general versus local anesthesia may potentially affect outcomes. Traditionally, IA cerebral interventional therapies have been performed under general anesthesia for patient safety. However, recent data have questioned this practice in the setting of intervention for acute ischemic stroke. The largest study was from a multicenter retrospective study of 980 patients undergoing IA therapy, 44% of whom were treated under general anesthesia.[32] This study showed that use of general anesthesia was associated with 2.33 odds ratio (95% confidence interval, 1.63–3.44; $P<.0001$) of poor outcome at 90 days and an odds ratio of death of 1.68 (95% confidence interval, 1.23–2.30; $P<.0001$). Similar negative results were noted in a retrospective analysis of 75 patients from the IMS II study that showed that patients treated with lesser degrees of anesthesia fared better with improved neurologic outcomes and lower mortality.[33] More recently, in the NASA Registry of patients with acute ischemic stroke treated with the Solitaire FR device, the use of general anesthesia was associated with worse neurologic outcomes and increased mortality.[34] The differences were clinically significant with a 40% higher probability of a good clinical outcome in those treated without general anesthesia and a three-fold lower risk of death.

Endovascular Interventions

Intra-arterial fibrinolysis

With the advent of mechanical interventional devices, the use of fibrinolytics in this setting has fallen drastically. This is particularly true with the most recent technological advances that have led to the approval of stent retrievers and aspiration catheters that have high recanalization efficacy. Furthermore, it is not uncommon for patients undergoing intervention for ischemic stroke to have already received IV tPA, making infusion of additional IA fibrinolytic a rather undesirable strategy compared with use of mechanical devices.

The procedure for delivering IA thrombolytics is simple compared with mechanical devices that do require significantly more technical expertise. Typically, the procedure involves placement of a guidecatheter (5F or 6F) in the vessel in question, usually the cervical internal carotid artery or the common carotid artery in the anterior circulation and the cervical vertebral artery in the posterior circulation. Then coaxially through the guidecatheter a microcatheter is advanced to the site of occlusion for delivery of the fibrinolytic drug. The position of the microcatheter for delivery of the drug is largely based on the preference of the operator. There is no standard guidance regarding position of the microcatheter, or IA drug dose delivered. Most centers tend to follow the dosage regimen used in the IMS trials. This had been the regimen used in EMS and the three IMS studies with acceptable rates of symptomatic hemorrhage,[6,7,15,16] although some centers have shown that higher doses may be safe.[35] In addition, in terms of choice of agent, there are no FDA-approved fibrinolytics for IA delivery, and hence most centers use tPA (ie, off-label use of a drug approved for IV use ischemic stroke).

The protocol in IMS III consists of initially placing the microcatheter distal to the thrombus with delivery of 1 mg of rtPA in this location. The microcatheter is then retracted just proximal into the proximal thrombus and an additional 1 mg of rtPA is hand injected, immediately followed by infusion at the rate of 10 mg/h for 2 hours. Frequent angiographic assessment, typically every 15 minutes, is performed, and once adequate recanalization is achieved, the infusion is stopped. A maximum IA dose of 22 mg is typically administered.

There are no standard recommended techniques for IA delivery of thrombolytics. In PROACT, the protocol was significantly different, with the infusion microcatheter placed into the proximal one-third of the middle cerebral artery thrombus with no mechanical disruption of the clot permitted.[10] After 1 hour of infusion, another angiogram was performed and if any of the proximal thrombus had dissolved, the interventionalist advanced the microcatheter tip into the proximal portion of any remaining clot in the middle cerebral artery and continued infusion.

The Merci retrieval technique

The Merci Retrieval System consists of the Merci Retriever, the Merci Balloon Guide Catheter (BGC), and the Merci microcatheter. The BGC is a 9F or 8F catheter with a balloon located at its distal tip. The Merci Retriever is made of memory-shaped nitinol (nickel titanium) and is a helical wire with the initial design consisting of five loops of decreasing diameter, from 2.8 to 1.1 mm at its distal end. The last generation of the Merci Retrievers consisted of five helical loops of the same diameter including a 2-, 2.5-, and 3.0-mm device to be used in appropriate sized vessel. Typically the 2-mm device was used in the M2 segment of the middle cerebral artery, 2.5 mm in M1, and 3.0 mm in the internal carotid artery.

The technique involves placing the BGC into the common or internal carotid artery for anterior circulation occlusions, or the subclavian artery (or vertebral artery if large enough) for posterior circulation occlusions. Using standard cerebral catheterization techniques, the microcatheter is guided into the occluded vessel and passed beyond the thrombus. A selective angiogram is performed distal to the thrombus to evaluate the size and tortuosity of the distal arteries and to confirm appropriate anatomy for deployment of the Merci Retriever. The Merci Retriever is then advanced through the microcatheter and fully deployed beyond the clot. The BGC balloon is inflated to arrest antegrade flow during removal of the thrombus. The Merci Retriever with the ensnared thrombus, and the microcatheter, are withdrawn together into the BGC lumen. Continuous aspiration is applied to the BGC to ensure complete evacuation of the thrombus. The balloon of the BGC is then deflated to re-establish blood flow and a repeat angiogram is performed. If the occlusion persists, the procedure is repeated up to six passes of the Merci Retriever.

Several aspects of this technique deserve mention. First, the Merci technique evolved as operators had more experience with the device and the previously described protocol for deployment of the Merci device is the latest technique that was used in this procedure. Second, the use of the BGC is not consistent among physicians, with some preferring a regular guidecatheter in lieu of the BGC. Those that insisted on the use of the BGC contend that it reduces the chances of clot fragmentation and distal embolization during retrieval.

Penumbra aspiration technique
The Penumbra System is an endovascular mechanical thrombectomy device that uses continuous aspiration to perform recanalization of occluded intracranial vessels. It uses a unique microcatheter and separator based thrombus debulking approach to intracranial revascularization. The system works by advancing a reperfusion catheter (the aspiration catheter) over a neurovascular guidewire until it reaches the occluding thrombus. The tip of the catheter is placed just proximal to the clot. An appropriately sized separator device is then introduced into the proximal part of the thrombus through the reperfusion catheter. The reperfusion catheter is then attached to an aspirator pump and the thrombus is effectively vacuumed from the blocked vessel while the separator is alternately advanced and retracted within the reperfusion catheter to aid with the extraction. There are variable size aspiration catheters available for different sized blood vessels.

Stent retrieval technique
The technique for stent retrieval of clots is essentially identical to that of the Merci procedure. The technique similarly involves placing a BGC into cervical internal carotid artery or the common carotid artery for anterior circulation occlusion, or the subclavian artery or vertebral artery for posterior circulation retrieval. The microcatheter is then guided into the occluded vessel and passed beyond the thrombus followed by a selective angiogram distal to the clot to evaluate and confirm the appropriate landing zone for the stent retriever. The stent retriever is then advanced through the microcatheter and unsheathed to capture the clot within the central portion of the device so that the device can fully expand within the clot and capture

it. The metal strands of the stent retriever allow multiple points of contact with the clot, and perhaps better engagement and entrapment of the clot within the device. The BGC balloon is inflated to arrest antegrade flow during removal of the thrombus just as in the Merci technique. The device is then withdrawn along with the ensnared thrombus and the microcatheter into the BGC lumen. Continuous aspiration is applied to the BGC to ensure that any particulate matter that is left behind in the vessel is adequately aspirated before deflation of the balloon, which re-establishes antegrade flow. A repeat angiogram is performed and if the occlusion persists, the procedure is repeated. The device is approved for up to three passes, although in practice physicians have performed up to six passes with the stent retrievers as was standard practice with the Merci device.

In the discussion with the Merci technique, the use of the BGC is controversial and many practitioners see this as an unnecessary step and use a standard guidecatheter in lieu of the BGC. Data, however, seem to indicate that the use of a BGC does indeed reduce the incidence of distal embolization, particularly into previously uninvolved territories, and may improve outcomes. In a recent prospective registry of patients with acute ischemic stroke treated with the Solitaire FR device, the use of a BGC seemed to improve recanalization rates, reduce distal embolizations, and increase rates of good outcomes.[36] Procedure time was shorter in patients with a BGC (120 $\pm$ 28.5 vs 161 $\pm$ 35.6 minutes; $P = .02$), and less adjunctive therapy was used in patients with a BGC (20% vs 28.6%; $P = .05$). TICI3 reperfusion scores were higher in patients with BGC use (53.7% vs 32.5%; $P<.001$). Distal emboli and emboli in new territory were similar between the two groups. Discharge NIHSS score (mean, 12 $\pm$ 14.5 vs 17.5 $\pm$ 16; $P = .002$) and good clinical outcome at 3 months were superior in patients with BGC compared with patients without (51.6% vs 35.8%; $P = .02$). Multivariate analysis demonstrated that the use of a BGC was an independent predictor of good clinical outcome (odds ratio, 2.5; 95% confidence interval, 1.2–4.9). In conclusion, data seem to justify the use of a BGC with superior revascularization results, faster procedure times, decreased need for adjunctive therapy, and improved clinical outcome.

REFERENCES

1. Tissue plasminogen activator for acute ischemic stroke. The National Institute of Neurologic Disorders and Stroke rt-PA Stroke Study Group. N Engl J Med 1995; 333:1581–7.
2. Hacke W, Kaste M, Bluhmki E, et al. Thrombolysis with alteplase 3 to 4.5 hours after acute ischemic stroke. N Engl J Med 2008;359:1317–29.
3. Lees KR, Bluhmki E, von Kummer R, et al. Time to treatment with intravenous alteplase and outcome in stroke: an updated pooled analysis of ECASS, ATLANTIS, NINDS, and EPITHET trials. Lancet 2010;375:1695–703.
4. Zeumer H, Hacke W, Ringelstein EB. Local intraarterial thrombolysis in vertebro-basilar thromboembolic disease. AJNR Am J Neuroradiol 1983;4:401–4.
5. del Zoppo GJ, Ferbert A, Otis S, et al. Local intra-arterial fibrinolytic therapy in acute carotid territory stroke. A pilot study. Stroke 1988;19:307–13.
6. Lewandowski CA, Frankel M, Tomsick TA, et al. Combined intravenous and intra-arterial r-tPA versus intra-arterial therapy of acute ischemic stroke: emergency management of stroke (EMS) bridging trial. Stroke 1999;30: 2598–605.
7. Broderick JP, Palesch YY, Demchuk AM, et al. Endovascular therapy after intravenous t-PA versus t-PA alone for stroke. N Engl J Med 2013;368:893–903.

8. Kidwell CS, Jahan R, Gornbein J, et al. A trial of imaging selection and endovascular treatment for ischemic stroke. N Engl J Med 2013;368:914–23.
9. Ciccone A, Valvassori L, Investigators SE. Endovascular treatment for acute ischemic stroke. N Engl J Med 2013;368:2433–4.
10. Furlan A, Higashida R, Wechsler L, et al. Intra-arterial prourokinase for acute ischemic stroke. The PROACT II study: a randomized controlled trial. Prolyse in acute cerebral thromboembolism. JAMA 1999;282:2003–11.
11. Ogawa A, Mori E, Minematsu K, et al. Randomized trial of intraarterial infusion of urokinase within 6 hours of middle cerebral artery stroke: the middle cerebral artery embolism local fibrinolytic intervention trial (MELT) Japan. Stroke 2007; 38:2633–9.
12. Gobin YP, Starkman S, Duckwiler GR, et al. Merci 1: a phase 1 study of mechanical embolus removal in cerebral ischemia. Stroke 2004;35:2848–54.
13. Smith WS, Sung G, Starkman S, et al. Safety and efficacy of mechanical embolectomy in acute ischemic stroke: results of the Merci trial. Stroke 2005;36: 1432–8.
14. Smith WS, Sung G, Saver J, et al. Mechanical thrombectomy for acute ischemic stroke: final results of the multi Merci trial. Stroke 2008;39:1205–12.
15. IMS Study Investigators. Combined intravenous and intra-arterial recanalization for acute ischemic stroke: the interventional management of stroke study. Stroke 2004;35:904–11.
16. IMS II Trial Investigators. The interventional management of stroke (IMS) II study. Stroke 2007;38:2127–35.
17. Khatri P, Abruzzo T, Yeatts SD, et al. Good clinical outcome after ischemic stroke with successful revascularization is time-dependent. Neurology 2009;73: 1066–72.
18. Khatri P, Yeatts SD, Mazighi M, et al. Time to angiographic reperfusion and clinical outcome after acute ischaemic stroke: an analysis of data from the interventional management of stroke (IMS III) phase 3 trial. Lancet Neurol 2014;13: 567–74.
19. Penumbra Pivotal Stroke Trial Investigators. The penumbra pivotal stroke trial: safety and effectiveness of a new generation of mechanical devices for clot removal in intracranial large vessel occlusive disease. Stroke 2009;40:2761–8.
20. Goyal M, Menon BK, Coutts SB, et al, Penumbra Pivotal Stroke Trial Investigators, Calgary Stroke Program. Effect of baseline CT scan appearance and time to recanalization on clinical outcomes in endovascular thrombectomy of acute ischemic strokes. Stroke 2011;42:93–7.
21. Saver JL, Jahan R, Levy EI, et al. Solitaire flow restoration device versus the Merci retriever in patients with acute ischaemic stroke (SWIFT): a randomised, parallel-group, non-inferiority trial. Lancet 2012;380:1241–9.
22. Nogueira RG, Lutsep HL, Gupta R, et al. Trevo versus Merci retrievers for thrombectomy revascularisation of large vessel occlusions in acute ischaemic stroke (TREVO 2): a randomised trial. Lancet 2012;380:1231–40.
23. Fransen PS, Beumer D, Berkhemer OA, et al. Mr clean, a multicenter randomized clinical trial of endovascular treatment for acute ischemic stroke in the Netherlands: study protocol for a randomized controlled trial. Trials 2014;15:343.
24. Kidwell CS, Wintermark M, De Silva DA, et al. Multiparametric MRI and CT models of infarct core and favorable penumbral imaging patterns in acute ischemic stroke. Stroke 2013;44:73–9.
25. Chimowitz MI. Endovascular treatment for acute ischemic stroke: still unproven. N Engl J Med 2013;368:952–5.

26. Ciccone A, Valvassori L, Nichelatti M, et al. Endovascular treatment for acute ischemic stroke. N Engl J Med 2013;368:904–13.
27. Kidwell CS. MRI biomarkers in acute ischemic stroke: a conceptual framework and historical analysis. Stroke 2013;44:570–8.
28. Olivot JM, Mlynash M, Thijs VN, et al. Optimal tmax threshold for predicting penumbral tissue in acute stroke. Stroke 2009;40:469–75.
29. Lansberg MG, Straka M, Kemp S, et al. MRI profile and response to endovascular reperfusion after stroke (defuse 2): a prospective cohort study. Lancet Neurol 2012;11:860–7.
30. Schonewille WJ, Wijman CA, Michel P, et al. Treatment and outcomes of acute basilar artery occlusion in the basilar artery international cooperation study (basics): a prospective registry study. Lancet Neurol 2009;8:724–30.
31. del Zoppo GJ, Higashida RT, Furlan AJ, et al. Proact: a phase ii randomized trial of recombinant pro-urokinase by direct arterial delivery in acute middle cerebral artery stroke. Proact investigators. Prolyse in acute cerebral thromboembolism. Stroke 1998;29:4–11.
32. Abou-Chebl A, Lin R, Hussain MS, et al. Conscious sedation versus general anesthesia during endovascular therapy for acute anterior circulation stroke: preliminary results from a retrospective, multicenter study. Stroke 2010;41: 1175–9.
33. Nichols C, Carrozzella J, Yeatts S, et al. Is peri-procedural sedation during acute stroke therapy associated with poorer functional outcomes? J Neurointerv Surg 2010;2:67–70.
34. Abou-Chebl A, Zaidat OO, Castonguay AC, et al. North American Solitaire Stent-Retriever Acute Stroke Registry: choice of anesthesia and outcomes. Stroke 2014;45:1396–401.
35. Qureshi AI, Suri MF, Shatla AA, et al. Intraarterial recombinant tissue plasminogen activator for ischemic stroke: an accelerating dosing regimen [in process citation]. Neurosurgery 2000;47:473–6 [discussion: 477–9].
36. Nguyen TN, Malisch T, Castonguay AC, et al. Balloon guide catheter improves revascularization and clinical outcomes with the solitaire device: analysis of the North American Solitaire Acute Stroke Registry. Stroke 2014;45:141–5.

Diagnosis and Treatment of Cervical Artery Dissection

Stefan T. Engelter, MD[a,b,*], Christopher Traenka, MD[a],
Alexander Von Hessling, MD[c], Philippe A. Lyrer, MD[a]

KEYWORDS

- Cervical artery dissection • Stroke • IV thrombolysis • Antipatelets • Anticoagulants
- Endovascular treatment • Surgery

KEY POINTS

- Cervical artery dissection (CAD) accounts for 2% to 2.5% of all ischemic strokes but is held responsible for 10% to 25% of all ischemic strokes in the young.
- In most patients, CAD is confirmed by visualization of a mural hematoma. MRI has a higher sensitivity than neurosonology but can be falsely negative in the first days.
- The intramural blood accumulation should not be considered a reason to withhold intravenous (IV) thrombolysis (IVT) in patients with acute ischemic stroke associated with CAD.
- Acute endovascular treatment has been shown feasible and might be an alternative to IVT alone; it is worthwhile studying in more detail.
- Antiplatelets and anticoagulants are used to prevent stroke in CAD patients and the findings of 4 large meta-analyses across observational data do not suggest any superiority of either treatment approach.
- Three randomized controlled trials (RCTs) compare anticoagulation versus antiplatelets in CAD, and participation is encouraged to increase the level of therapeutic evidence.
- Angioplasty and stenting are usually reserved for CAD patients with recurrent ischemic events despite antithrombotic therapy, when hemodynamic infarction is impending, in ruptured dissecting aneurysm or in iatrogenic CAD.
- Surgery is limited mostly to CAD patients with a progressive clinical course despite medical treatment, with anatomically accessible lesions, and in whom there are arguments against stenting.

Disclosures: The work on this review was supported by the Basel Stroke-Funds and grants of the Swiss National Science Foundation (33CM30-124119; 33CM30-140340/1) and of the Swiss Heart Foundation. The authors are investigators of the TREAT-CAD study.
[a] Department of Neurology and Stroke Center, University Hospital Basel, Petersgraben 4, Basel CH – 4031, Switzerland; [b] Neurorehabilitation Unit, Felix Platter Hospital, University Center for Medicine of Aging and Rehabilitation, Burgfelderstrasse 101, Basel CH – 4012, Switzerland; [c] Department of Radiology, Neuroradiology and Stroke Center, University Hospital Basel, Petersgraben 4, Basel CH – 4031, Switzerland
* Corresponding author. Department of Neurology and Stroke Center, University Hospital Basel, Petersgraben 4, Basel CH – 4031, Switzerland.
E-mail address: stefan.engelter@usb.ch

0733-8619/15/$ – see front matter © 2015 Elsevier Inc. All rights reserved.

EPIDEMIOLOGY AND SIGNIFICANCE

Cervical artery dissection (CAD) is characterized by an intramural hematoma of the internal carotid artery or the vertebral artery.[1–3] CAD generally accounts for 2% to 2.5% of all ischemic strokes.[4] Depending on the definition of *young*, however, CAD is responsible for 10% to 25% of all ischemic strokes in younger-aged patients[1] and is considered a major cause of stroke.[3,5] The incidence has been reported to be 2.6 to 3.0 per 100.000 inhabitants per year.[6,7] For extracranial internal carotid artery dissection (ICAD) and extracranial vertebral artery dissection (VAD), the incidence was found 1.7 to 3.0/100 000 and 0.97 (95% CI, 0.52–1.4) per 100,000 per year, respectively.[6–9] These figures indicate that extracranial ICAD can be expected twice as often as extracranial VAD.[6] The Cervical Artery Dissection and Ischemic Stroke Patients (CADISP) study, a multinational registry across 18, mostly European, centers, included all consecutive patients with a diagnosis of CAD presenting with stroke, transient ischemic attack (TIA), or nonischemic symptoms.[10] In this study population, ICAD (n = 619) was more common than VAD (n = 327).[11] In turn, according to the observations of the Canadian Stroke Consortium, VAD was even more common than ICAD.[12] This observation was confirmed by a recent epidemiologic study from Dijon, France, that revealed incidence rates of 1.21/100 000 per year and 1.87/100 000 per year for ICAD and VAD, respectively. This study, however, included only patients with stroke or TIA attributable to CAD.[7]

The average age of CAD patients is approximately 45 years.[7,11,13–16] When experiencing CAD, men are on average 5 years older than women. CAD in general is slightly more common in men (52%–69%) than in women.[7,8,14,17–19] Compared with VAD, the dissection of internal carotid artery shows a slight preference for male and older patients.[11,16]

PATHOPHYSIOLOGY

The pathophysiologic hallmark of CAD is an intramural hematoma, which is thought caused by a subintimal tear into the arterial wall of the carotid or the vertebral artery. The mural blood accumulation can be located subadventitially—thereby, it may cause local compression syndromes (eg, Horner syndrome) or, in cases of arterial rupture, may result in a subarachnoid hemorrhage, the latter more frequent in intracranial than in extracranial dissections. Moreover, the intramural hematoma can lead to arterial narrowing, causing stenosis or vessel occlusion and yielding cerebral ischemic events. Originating from the injured intima, these cerebral ischemic events are more often embolic rather than due to hemodynamic compromise.[20]

CLINICAL PRESENTATION AND DIAGNOSIS

CADs may become clinically apparent as stroke or TIA, which is the case in approximately two-thirds of all CAD patients. Often clinical presentation is a combination of ischemic events and local symptoms (Horner syndrome, cranial nerve palsy, tinnitus, or cervical root impairment).[21,22] In addition, these symptoms are often associated with headache or neck pain.[22] If CAD is suspected, a diagnosis of CAD is confirmed by the presence of at least 1 of the following neurovascular criteria: visualization of a mural hematoma, aneurysmal dilatation, long tapering stenosis, intimal flap, double lumen, and occlusion greater than 2 cm above the carotid bifurcation revealing an aneurysmal dilatation or a long tapering stenosis after recanalization in the internal carotid or vertebral artery.[23,24]

These imaging features are most accurately visualized by MRI, with identification of mural hematoma by fat-suppressed T1 sequences (**Fig. 1**). Yet, visualization of characteristic features of CAD by CT or neurosonography is also possible (**Fig. 2**).[25] Compared with MRI, neurosonography has a lower sensitivity in the diagnosis of CAD. Although in MRI the detection of mural hematoma can be falsely negative in the very acute stage, neurosonography may depict CAD characteristics, including mural hematoma, even early after CAD onset.[26]

THERAPEUTIC DILEMMA

CAD is characterized by a mural bleed. In theory, IVT—and to a lesser extent also anticoagulation—might promote extension of the intramural bleeding, which may lead to a progressive hemodynamic worsening and infarct growth.[27] Thus, with regard to therapeutic decisions, it is debated whether (1) IVT is the treatment of choice in patients with acute ischemic stroke attributable to CAD and (2) anticoagulation is superior to antiplatelets in CAD treatment.

INTRAVENOUS THROMBOLYSIS IN CERVICAL ARTERY DISSECTION

In patients treated with IVT for myocardial infarction, IVT has been shown harmful and dangerous in the presence of aortic dissection.[28,29] In patients suffering from acute ischemic stroke, IVT is beneficial independent of underlying stroke cause. Although it is questionable if this includes in particular stroke attributable to CAD, there are arguments in favor of IVT: IVT in CAD can be beneficial by inducing recanalization of the arterial thrombosis at the site of dissection or of a distal embolus.[27] A recent

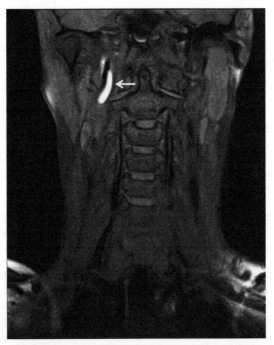

Fig. 1. MRI showing mural hematoma of the right internal carotid artery. Fat-suppressed T1-weighted image with high signal intensity indicating mural hematoma (*arrow*).

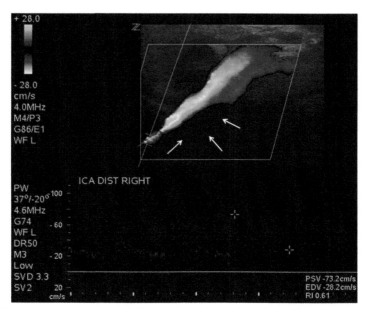

Fig. 2. Neurosonology with mural hematoma of the right internal carotid artery (same patient as in **Fig. 1**, 4 hours earlier). Duplex sonography of the distal internal carotid artery on the right shows (1) hypoechogenicity of the arterial wall (*arrows*), which leads to (2) a lumen narrowing, and (3) a mild alias phenomenon.

case report showed that even in a tandem occlusion due to CAD, IVT can be beneficial.[30]

INTRAVENOUS THROMBOLYSIS IN CERVICAL ARTERY DISSECTION PATIENTS VERSUS NON–CERVICAL ARTERY DISSECTION PATIENTS

There are no data on IVT in CAD from RCTs. In this situation, data from observational cohort studies is helpful to put impressions from individual case experiences into perspective.

Among 1062 IVT-treated Swiss stroke patients, subjects with stroke related to CAD (n = 55) were compared with subjects with stroke cause other than CAD (n = 1007).[24] In this population, only 36% (20/55) of all CAD patients receiving IVT had an excellent outcome compared with 44% (447/1007) of all non-CAD patients treated with IVT. Excellent outcome in this study was defined as modified Rankin scale (mRS) score 0 or 1 at 3 months. This lower recovery rate of CAD patients was significant after adjustment for age, gender, and stroke severity (odds ratio [OR] 0.50 [95% CI, 0.27–0.95]; P = .03). Neither differences in the rate of intracranial hemorrhages (ICHs) (symptomatic ICH in 5% within each group) nor the frequency of recurrent ischemic stroke (1.8% [CAD] vs 3.7% [non-CAD]) are explanatory for the worse outcome results of the CAD patients. Hence, these findings suggest a less favorable recovery of CAD patients after IVT. A possible explanation is the high rate of large artery occlusion observed in CAD patients (67.7%).[27] Taking into account that larger artery occlusion in general is a known negative prognostic factor in IVT,[31] these data may also suggest that an endovascular approach could be superior to IVT alone.

Most recently, a meta-analysis reported on the outcome of 121 IV-thrombolyzed and 59 intra-arterial–thrombolyzed CAD patients across 14 retrospective series and

22 case reports and provided a comparison with age- and stroke severity–matched patients from the Safe Implementation of Thrombolysis in Stroke-International Stroke Thrombolysis Register (SITS-ISTR).[32,33]

Thrombolyzed CAD patients had severe strokes, indicated by a median National Institutes of Health Stroke Scale (NIHSS) score of 16. At the end of a median follow-up period of 3 months (range 5 days–180 days), 33.3% (95% CI, 25.5–42.2) of the IVT group reached an mRS score of 0 to 1, and 60.8% (96% CI, 51.8–69.1) of this group reached an mRS score of 0 to 2. Those IV-thrombolyzed CAD patients, for whom comparisons with matched patients with all-stroke causes from SITS-ISTR were feasible, had rates for all endpoints similar to the comparison group, with largely overlapping 95% CIs. These endpoints included 3-month mortality (7.3% [3.7–13.9] vs 8.8% [5.1–14.5]), symptomatic ICH (3.3% [1.2–8.5] vs 5.9% [3.0–10.9]), and excellent 3-month outcome (mRS 0–1) (30.9% [23.0–40.1] vs 37.4% [30.3–45.8]). Thus, in this study, safety and outcome measures of IVT in patients with CAD-associated stroke seemed similar to those for IVT in patients with stroke due to all causes.[33]

THROMBOLYSIS VERSUS NONTHROMBOLYSIS IN CERVICAL ARTERY DISSECTION

Current treatment guidelines do not recommend against IVT treatment in CAD patients, although there are no data from RCTs on IVT versus placebo in such patients. There are nonrandomized comparisons of CAD patients treated with thrombolysis for ischemic stroke versus those treated without. In a small pilot trial, 7 patients with ICAD treated with IVT tended toward a worse outcome than 7 patients who did not receive IVT. Yet the sample size disallowed adjustments for potential confounders.[34]

Furthermore, based on the CADISP registry, 68 (11.0%) CAD patients receiving thrombolysis were compared with 548 CAD patients treated without thrombolysis. After adjustment for confounding variables (ie, stroke severity and vessel occlusion), the chance to recover favorably was virtually identical for IVT- and non-IVT–treated CAD patients (adjusted OR 0.95 [95% CI, 0.45–2.00]). The same finding was obtained by using a propensity matching score model with an OR of 1.00 (0.49–2.00) for a 3-month mRS score of 0 to 2.

In absolute terms, more than half of the thrombolyzed CAD patients reached a favorable outcome (ie, mRS 0–2 after 3 months).[27] Similar rates were obtained in smaller series (3/6[35], 4/11[36], 3/7[23], and 17/33[37]) and the meta-analysis (discussed previously) across retrospective cases, which reported 58.2% (48.8–67.0) of patients who reached an mRS score of 0 to 2.[33] Furthermore, this rate is similar to those reported in the RCTs on IVT in acute ischemic stroke patients[38,39] and the SITS-ISTR registry of IVT for stroke of miscellaneous causes.[32]

Symptomatic ICHs as well as major extracranial hemorrhages were absent, and asymptomatic ICHs occurred in only 5.9% of the thrombolyzed CAD patients.[27] This rate was lower than reported in the *National Institute of Neurological Disorders and Stroke* and the European Cooperative Acute Stroke Study III studies adhering to the same definitions.[38,39]

For comparison, among the nonthrombolyzed CAD patients, 3 (0.6%) patients had major hemorrhages. These include asymptomatic ICH (n = 2) and major extracranial hemorrhage (n = 1). Such data suggest a certain safety of thrombolysis in CAD patients with regard to relevant bleeding complications.[27]

ACUTE ENDOVASCULAR RECANALIZATION THERAPY

There are case reports and small series of acute endovascular treatment in acute ischemic stroke related to CAD.[40–44] Patients with occlusion of the dissected extracranial artery and occlusion of a main segment of a large intracranial artery were also treated.[41] Some of these patients had IVT followed by endovascular treatments, including intra-arterial thrombolysis as well as mechanical revascularization with or without stenting. These reports show the feasibility of this approach, although there is a certain risk that the false lumen might be chosen for recanalization procedures. Furthermore, intraluminal thrombus in the dissected carotid artery is considered a contraindication for stenting.[41] The authors performed a meta-analysis across 5 non-randomized observational case series in which a total of 111 patients were treated with either IVT alone or acute endovascular treatment.[23,27,40,42,43] The OR of 1.41 (95% CI, 0.45–3.45) indicates neither an advantage nor any harm of the acute endovascular approach (**Table 1**). Data were not adjusted, however, for confounding variables, such as stroke severity.

Another large meta-analysis of retrospective series and case reports included 59 CAD patients treated with acute endovascular treatment; 121 patients treated with IVT served as reference. Adjusted for stroke severity, the ORs were 1.66 (0.80–3.43) for excellent outcome (mRS 0–1) and 1.45 (0.61–3.45) for favorable outcome (mRS 0–2).[33] The point estimate of the OR might suggest that acute endovascular treatment has the potential for superiority compared with IV thrombolysis. The large 95% CIs, however, and several methodological limitations urge a cautious interpretation of this finding. Furthermore, in recent RCTs of stroke of miscellaneous causes, the acute endovascular treatment failed to show superiority to IVT alone.[45]

In conclusion, despite theoretic concerns about using thrombolysis in CAD patients, the available clinical evidence shows safety and certain effectiveness, indicating that thrombolysis in these patients should not be withheld. It remains unclear, however, whether such patients should be treated with IVT or whether acute endovascular treatment is a useful alternative option, in particular in CAD patients with intracranial occlusions or tandem occlusions.

SUMMARY OF ARGUMENTS AND COUNTERARGUMENTS FOR THE PREFERENCE OF INTRAVENOUS THROMBOLYSIS IN CERVICAL ARTERY DISSECTION PATIENTS

IV thrombolysis is the treatment of choice in acute ischemic stroke attributable to CAD

1. IV thrombolysis has been reported beneficial in acute ischemic stroke independently of the underlying etiology. (Category T1, level of clinical efficacy 1-1).
2. IV thrombolysis can induce recanalization of an arterial thrombosis in stroke attributable to CAD as well as in the more frequent other causes of stroke such as cardioembolism or large-artery atherosclerosis. (Category T4, Level of clinical efficacy U).
3. In case series and explorative clinical studies, IV thrombolysis in CAD patients was neither associated with increased mortality, nor in an excess of symptomatic bleedings nor more recurrent ischemic strokes. Thus, safety of IVT in CAD-related stroke appears similar to those for stroke from other causes. (Category T4, Level of clinical efficacy U).
4. Functional outcome in thrombolyzed patients with CAD-related stroke appear similar to that in stroke from all causes in the large thrombolysis RCTs and a large European thrombolysis registry. (Category T4, Level of clinical efficacy U).
5. There is no evidence that endovascular treatment is superior to IV treatment in CAD. (Category T4, Level of clinical efficacy U).

Table 1

Intravenous thrombolysis versus acute endovascular treatment in cervical artery dissection with regard to favorable outcome; meta-analysis across observational cases series comparing both treatment options

Study or Subgroup	Intravenous Thrombolysis		Endovascular		Weight	Peto Odds Ratio Peto, Fixed (95% CI)	Peto Odds Ratio Peto, Fixed (95% CI)
	Events	Total	Events	Total			
Lavallée,[40] 2008	1	4	4	6	13.9%	0.22 (0.02, 2.46)	
Baumgartner,[42] 2008	6	14	2	4	17.0%	0.76 (0.09, 6.69)	
Arnold,[23] 2002	1	2	3	7	9.0%	1.29 (0.07, 25.50)	
Engelter (CADISP),[27] 2012	32	55	5	13	55.4%	2.19 (0.66, 7.30)	
Vergouwen,[43] 2009	4	4	1	2	4.6%	20.09 (0.31, 1283.97)	
Total (95% CI)		79		32	100.0%	1.41 (0.57, 3.45)	
Total events	44		15				

Forest plot axis: 0.001 — 0.1 — 1 — 10 — 1000; Endovascular therapy ← → IV Thrombolysis

Heterogeneity: $\chi^2 = 4.66$, $df = 4$ ($P = .32$); $I^2 = 14\%$.
Test for overall effect: $z = 0.75$ ($P = .46$).

INTRAVENOUS THROMBOLYSIS IS NOT THE TREATMENT OF CHOICE IN ALL PATIENTS WITH ACUTE ISCHEMIC STROKE DUE TO CERVICAL ARTERY DISSECTION

1. Observational findings suggest that patients with CAD-related stroke benefit less from IVT than those with stroke attributable to other causes (category T4, level of clinical efficacy U).
2. The lower recovery rate, observed in some studies, could be due to a high rate of mechanical arterial occlusion (by the intimal flap and mural hematoma) and further distal thromboembolism with tandem occlusion. This feature might respond better to endovascular recanalization than to IVT (category T4, level of clinical efficacy U).
3. The available data on acute endovascular treatment in CAD—including mechanical revascularization—indicate the legitimacy of studying whether or not this approach is a treatment option that is at least as efficient as IVT (category T4, level of clinical efficacy U).

RECURRENT ISCHEMIC EVENT

Some prospective studies suggest a high early risk of recurrent stroke in CAD patients.[12,46] The cumulative recurrent stroke rate during the first year was 10.7% (95% CI, 6.5%–14.9%),[46] whereas 5.2% of the patients experienced their recurrent event during hospitalization. Beletsky and colleagues[12] reported a recurrence rate of stroke or TIA as high as 13.3% within 1 year of follow-up. Such numbers were not consistent, however, with further studies reporting lower stroke rates of 1.7% in patients treated with antiplatelets and 3.57% of patients treated with anticoagulants.[4,11,47] Most recurrent strokes occurred within 2 weeks after symptom onset of CAD.[48] Approximately 1 in 4 CAD patients had new ischemic lesions on diffusion-weighted imaging on follow-up MRI within 30 days.[49]

ANTITHROMBOTIC TREATMENT

In 2003, a systematic review reported on 3 of 91 (3.3%) CAD patients with "no antithrombotic therapy" who had a first or recurrent stroke during the follow-up period.[50] Lower rates of first or recurrent strokes in patients with antiplatelets (1.8%) or with anticoagulants (1.8%) were reported in the same review.[50] These differences, however, must not be considered a proof of beneficial effects of any type of antithrombotic treatment. Yet it may also reflect a bias, because "no antithrombotic therapy" might have been primarily applied for patients who were considered to have a poor prognosis.[50] Still, in consideration of the beneficial effect of antithrombotic agents in ischemic stroke in general, there is consensus to use antiplatelets or anticoagulants in all CAD patients in whom use of these agents is not contraindicated (eg, subarachnoid hemorrhage related to CAD).

Although there is consensus on the need for any antithrombotic treatment, there is equipoise regarding if CAD patients should be treated with anticoagulants or antiplatelets.[51] Most physicians still favor anticoagulants,[18,47,52] although it is unclear if anticoagulants are superior to antiplatelets, balancing risk and benefits of either approach.[53–55] Recurrent strokes occurred either way, under antiplatelets and under anticoagulants.[20,46]

META-ANALYSES OF OBSERVATIONAL DATA ON ANTIPLATELETS VERSUS ANTICOAGULATION

Four systematic meta-analyses comparing antiplatelets and anticoagulants in CAD patients have been performed.[47,48,56,57] In these meta-analyses, the 3-month mortality

rate ranged from 1.2% to 2.7%.[47,48,56,57] Menon and colleagues[56] reported no difference between antiplatelets and anticoagulants with regard to occurrence of stroke or
death. Lyrer and Engelter[48] observed a trend in favor of anticoagulants for "death or
disability" (P = .06), whereas, in turn, although rare, symptomatic ICHs (5/627;
0.8%) and major extracranial hemorrhages (7/425; 1.6%) occurred exclusively in the
anticoagulation group. Sarikaya and colleagues[57] showed a benefit of antiplatelets
compared with anticoagulants for preventing the composite outcome of ischemic
stroke, ICH, or death (relative risk 0.32; 95% credibility interval, 0.12–0.64). Kennedy
and colleagues[47] found no difference between antiplatelets and anticoagulants with
regard to risk of (1) recurrent stroke and (2) death. Details of the 4 meta-analyses
are summarized in **Table 2**.

These findings should be interpreted cautiously, because all meta-analyses had to
be based on observational data that are prone to bias.[48,57] Nevertheless, conclusions
based on these results can be helpful to generate hypotheses. In particular, these
meta-analyses support the idea that RCTs are ethically justified, medically required,
and widely advocated.[20,48,51,53,57]

RANDOMIZED CONTROLLED TRIALS

Currently there are 3 RCTs comparing antiplatelets to anticoagulants in CAD. The Cervical Artery Dissection in Stroke Study (CADISS) compares antiplatelets to anticoagulants in patients with CAD, which became clinically apparent within 7 days prior to
randomization. The primary outcome measure is ipsilateral stroke or death of all
causes within 3 months. The trial was designed to study feasibility. Specifically
CADISS aimed at exploring (1) whether there are sufficient clinical endpoints to provide the power to determine a treatment effect and (2) whether adequate numbers
of patients can be recruited (www.dissection.co.uk). The target number of 250 has
been reached and the study results are awaited.

The Pilot Study of Aspirin Versus Warfarin for Cervicocephalic Arterial Dissection
was planned as an RCT for a study population of 20 patients to be recruited between
March 2005 and March 2007. Unfortunately, the current status of recruitment is
unknown (www.clinicaltrials.gov/ct2/show/study/NCT00265408).

Estimates based on the meta-analyses (discussed previously) suggest that an RCT
based on pure clinical outcomes may be a huge venture because a large sample size
(n ≥2000) is required. Thus, surrogate outcome markers may be useful in this situation.
Diffusion-weighted MRI (DWI) is considered an ideal candidate as a surrogate marker
for ischemic events. An RCT testing surgery versus stenting in carotid stenosis
showed that the usage of DWI as (surrogate) outcome marker revealed the same
results as the clinical study—with approximately 10% of the patients.[58] Likewise, adding new silent microbleeds in MRI has been demonstrated to be useful as a surrogate
for ICH.[59]

Hence, using magnetic resonance surrogates, an open-labeled, multicenter,
noninferiority RCT comparing aspirin to anticoagulant treatment (vitamin K antagonists) in CAD patients with regard to outcome and complication measures has
been designed in Switzerland. The Biomarkers and Antithrombotic Treatment in
Cervical Artery Dissection (TREAT-CAD) study aims at demonstrating non-
inferiority of aspirin compared with vitamin K antagonists in CAD patients with regard to a composite outcome of clinical or imaging endpoints of brain ischemia,
bleeds, or death (NCT02046460 www.clinicaltrials.gov). TREAT-CAD has been
recruiting patients since September 2013. Details of all 3 RCTs are summarized
in **Table 3**.

Table 2
Synopsis of meta-analyses across observational data comparing antiplatelets with anticoagulants in cervical artery dissection

Author, Year	Site of Dissection	Methodology	Number of Patients	Main Results
Menon et al,[56] 2008	ICA, VA	Meta-analysis	762	No significant difference in risk of • Death: antiplatelet 5/268 (1.8%), anticoag. 9/494 (1.8%), $P = .88$ • Stroke: antiplatelet 5/268 (1.9%), anticoag.10/494 (2.0%), $P = .66$
Lyrer & Engelter,[48] 2010	ICA	Cochrane system. review	1285	Nonsignificant trend in favor of anticoagulants for • Death or disability (OR 1.77 [0.98 to 3.22],[a] $P = .06$) (463 patients) No significant differences in odds • Death (OR 2.02; 95% CI, 0.62–6.60) • Ischemic stroke (OR 0.63; 95% CI, 0.21–1.86) (1262 patients) Sympt. ICHs (5/627; 0.8%) only with anticoag. Major extracranial hemorrhages (7/425; 1.6%) only with anticoag.
Kennedy et al,[47] 2012	ICA, VA	Meta-analysis	1636	No significant differences in risk of • Restroke: antiplatelet 13/499 (2.6%), anticoag. 20/1137 (1.8%) • Death: antiplatelet 5/499 (1.0%), anticoag. 9/1137 (0.80%)
Sarikaya et al,[57] 2013	ICA, VA	Bayesian meta-analysis	1991	Antiplatelets lead significant reduction of composite outcome • Ischemic stroke, ICH, or death (3 mo) • Relative risk 0.32 (0.12 to 0.63)[b]

Abbreviations: Anticoag, anticoagulation; ICA, internal carotid artery; Sympt, symptomatic; System, systematic; VA, vertebral artery.
[a] 95% CI.
[b] 95% Credibility interval.

Table 3
Synopsis of randomized controlled trials comparing antiplatelets versus anticoagulants in cervical artery dissection

Study	Beginning	Type	Treatment	Primary Outcome	Target (Patients)	Current Status[a]	Recruited	ClinicalTrial.gov Identifier
CADISS	2005	Randomized controlled prospective multicenter study	Antiplatelets[b] vs anticoagulants	Ispilateral stroke or death within 3 mo from randomization	250	Recruitment completed	250	NCT 00238667
TREAT-CAD	2013	Randomized controlled open-label multicenter, noninferiority trial with blinded assessment of outcome events	Aspirin, 300 mg OD, vs vitamin K antagonists	Cerebrovascular ischemia, major hemorrhagic events, or death[c]	169	Recruiting	15	NCT 02046460
Jensen	2005	Randomized controlled open-label study	Aspirin vs warfarin	Stroke (1 y)	20	Unknown (last update 2007)	Unknown	NCT 00265408

[a] September 24, 2014.

[b] Antiplatelets: aspirin, dipyridamole, clopidogrel; anticoagulants: unfractionated heparin, dalteparin, enoxaparin, tinzaparin, warfarin.

[c] Primary outcome includes the following efficacy and safety outcome measures during the 3 month-treatment period: (1) occurrence of any stroke, new acute lesions on diffusion-weighted MRI (2) any major extracranial hemorrhage, any symptomatic intracranial hemorrhage and any asymptomatic micro-or macro bleeds, (3) death.

EMBOLIC SIGNALS IN TRANSCRANIAL DOPPLER MONITORING STUDIES

Transcranial Doppler (TCD) monitoring studies revealed microembolic signals (MESs) downstream of the dissected arteries. In ICAD, such signals were detected in the middle cerebral artery.[60–64] Similarly, in VAD, MESs were shown in the posterior cerebral artery.[60] The frequency of MESs in CAD patients is reported within the range of 25% to 60%.[60–64] MESs are detected more frequently in CAD patients presenting with stroke than in CAD patients with pure nonischemic signs or symptoms.[61] In addition, most CAD patients with recurrent ischemia have MESs (ie, 6/7[63] and 3/3[60]). These findings suggest that CAD patients with MESs may harbor an increased stroke risk than MES-negative CAD patients. Furthermore, these findings might indicate that ischemic events in CAD are mainly caused by embolism originating from the dissected artery. Such pathophysiologic considerations may serve as an argument in favor of a stronger antithrombotic therapy (ie, favoring anticoagulation over antiplatelets). MESs have been reported, however, in CAD patients independent from the type of antithrombotic treatment.[60,64] It is unclear if MESs occur more frequently in CAD patients treated with aspirin than in those treated with anticoagulation. Among a population of 20 CAD patients, all 5 MES-positive ones had some form of antithrombotic therapy during TCD monitoring—heparin in 3, aspirin in 1, and aspirin plus heparin in the remaining patient.[60] As a limitation, recording times in all patients were short, maybe too short to detect MESs in some patients who were considered MES negative.

In MESs originating from atherosclerotic carotid artery stenosis, cessation of MESs was associated with use of antiplatelets rather than with anticoagulants.[65] The Clopidogrel and Aspirin for Reduction of Emboli in Symptomatic Carotid Stenosis trial data showed that the combined antiplatelet therapy with aspirin plus clopidogrel reduced MESs in carotid stenosis of atherosclerotic origin.[66] Whether or not this can be translated into CAD patients remains unclear.

The significance of these observations is limited by (1) sample sizes of 6 to 28 patients, (2) the short TCD recording times, and (3) the nonrandomized allocation of treatment (aspirin or anticoagulation). Further studies have to prove if the presence of MESs identifies a subgroup of CAD patients at particular high risk of (recurrent) cerebral ischemia and—if treatment allocation was randomized—whether or not the presence or the number of MESs differs between CAD patients according to their antithrombotic treatment. Both the CADISS and the TREAT-CAD study have introduced TCD substudies. Thus, in the future, findings of the RCT substudies might clarify if MESs are useful to tailor the type of antithrombotic treatment in CAD.

ENLARGEMENTS OF THE MURAL HEMATOMA OVER TIME

The enlargement of the initial mural hematoma has been studied in a pilot study of 33 CAD patients; 17 (52%) experienced a growth of the mural hematoma over time. Because all patients had been treated with anticoagulants, however, it remained unclear if the observed hematoma enlargement was related to the treatment type or any treatment.[67]

More recently, the evolution of the mural hematoma in CAD during the first week after initiation of treatment with either antiplatelets (n = 13) or anticoagulation (n = 31) was studied by using dedicated cervical MRI of the arterial wall. Mean volumes of the mural hematoma decreased within 1 week after treatment onset by approximately 10% to 13% in both groups. One-third of all patients in each group, however, experienced some growth of the mural hematoma as well as an increase in length. Neither anticoagulation nor antiplatelet treatment was related to new ischemic events, worsening of existing deficits, or a reduction of the arterial lumen.[68] This is in contrast to case reports[25] or case series[69] that observed secondary carotid occlusion in 5 over-anticoagulated patients receiving heparin.[69] Although in most cases the occlusion remained asymptomatic, 1 patient developed a watershed infarction.[69] Although a relationship is suggestive, the clear evidence of an extended mural hematoma triggered by (over) anticoagulation was lacking. Furthermore, it remained unclear if the association between anticoagulation and delayed carotid occlusion was clearly causal and not coincidental. Bachmann and colleagues[70] reported on 24 dissected arteries, of which the degree of stenosis had increased in 2 (8%), remained unchanged in 13 (54%), and decreased in 9 (38%) arteries. These changes have been observed in follow-up high-resolution (3-T) MRI 2 weeks after baseline MRI.

In conclusion, based on the evidence in ischemic stroke in general, CAD patients should be treated with antithrombotic agents, in particular those who suffered from ischemic events due to CAD. Four meta-analyses of observational data showed no difference between both treatment approaches or differed in their suggestion of superiority depending on the chosen outcome measure. The question of superiority of either treatment can only be answered with data from RCTs, which are currently missing, although such trials are under way and participation is encouraged.

The reasoning in favor or against the use of anticoagulation in CAD can be based not only on the clinical studies (discussed previously) but also on pathophysiologic characteristics and considerations and conclusions by analogy, summarized as follows

ARGUMENTS FAVORING "ANTICOAGULATION IS SUPERIOR TO ANTIPLATELETS IN CERVICAL ARTERY DISSECTION PATIENTS"

1. The Cochrane systematic review reported nonsignificant superiority of anticoagulants over antiplatelets with regard to "death or disability" (category T4, level of clinical efficacy U).[48]
2. Another, at least theoretic, argument in favor of anticoagulation is the risk of clot formation in cases of arterial occlusion attributable to CAD. Cases of free-floating thrombi in dissected internal carotid arteries have been reported.[71] In addition, most occluded arteries recanalize over time, 30% within 8 days, and 60% to 80% within 3 months.[72,73] During the recanalization process, clots may be mobilized and transported downstream, where they can cause blockage of intracranial arteries prompting embolic infarctions[74] (category T4, level of clinical efficacy U).
3. Several arguments support an embolic mechanism, such as the observation of microemboli, the occurrence of distal branch occlusions and the infarct lesion pattern on brain scans. Conclusions by analogy to cardioembolic stroke (eg, due to atrial fibrillation), where anticoagulation is superior to antiplatelets (eg, aspirin) in secondary stroke prevention, these observations favor anticoagulation in stroke prevention of CAD. The assignability to CAD patients is, however, questionable. Conclusions by analogy from atherosclerotic carotid artery disease are limited due to the younger age and different pathomechanisms in CAD patients (category T4, level of clinical efficacy U).

ARGUMENTS FAVORING "ANTICOAGULATION IS NOT SUPERIOR TO ANTIPLATELETS IN CERVICAL ARTERY DISSECTION PATIENTS"

1. At least 1 meta-analysis reported that antiplatelets were superior to anticoagulants with regard to a composite outcome of "ischemic stroke, intracranial hemorrhage or death" (category T4, level of clinical efficacy U).[57]
2. In CAD patients with severe strokes, immediate anticoagulation may be potentially hazardous. This theoretic concern is based on findings of an increased rate of

symptomatic hemorrhagic transformation in severe strokes in the Trial of Org 10172 in Acute Stroke Treatment.[75] Applying the American Stroke Association guidelines for anticoagulation in stroke patients (2003)[76], immediate anticoagulation in CAD patients with NIHSS score of 15 or more cannot be recommended[76] (category T4, level of clinical efficacy U).

3. Although causality and clinical meaning are unclear, delayed occlusion of a dissected artery has been reported more often under anticoagulation than under antiplatelets[25,67–69] (category T4, level of clinical efficacy U).

If participation in an RCT is not feasible, it is recommended to base the decision on antithrombotic treatment in an individual CAD patient on empirical arguments. A synopsis of features in favor or against early anticoagulation in CAD is useful for decisions on a case-by-case basis (**Box 1**).

TREATMENT DURATION

There are no reliable data on the optimum duration of antithrombotic treatment in CAD. Yet, because the ideal duration of such a treatment has not been studied in clinical trials and is therefore unclear,[4] the duration of treatment has to be based on clinical reasoning taking into account the knowledge about the time course of (1) recurrent ischemic events, (2) recanalization, and (3) recurrent dissections. Most ischemic events occur within the first 2 weeks (discussed previously). Partial or complete recanalization of initial occlusion or high-grade stenosis in dissected carotid arteries occurs in 60% to 67% of all cases within 6 months after first onset of CAD.[72,73,77,78] Between 6 and 12 months after CAD onset, the recanalization rate is much lower at 6.8% and is only occurring in a few individual cases after 12 months.[78] The stroke rate in long-term follow-up of ICAD patients is not related to the persistence of carotid stenosis or occlusion.[79] The risk of recurrent dissection is also dropping considerably with the course of time: in 19% to 26%, a recurrent dissection in 1 of the previously nonaffected arteries may occur within 4 weeks according to some reports.[78,80] Thereafter, the risk of recurrence is declining to a rate between 3% and 6%.[74] The long-term risk for recurrent dissections is poorly known but possibly low, indicated by the finding of

---

Box 1
Empiric arguments to support antithrombotic treatment decisions on a case-by-case basis

Features: in favor of early anticoagulation

- MESs (transcranial neurosonology) despite ≥1 antiplatelets
- (Pseudo)occlusion of the dissected artery
- Multiple TIAs/strokes (same circulation)
- Free-floating thrombus

Features: against early anticoagulation → antiplatelets preferred

- Severe clinical deficit (NIHSS score ≥15).
- Accompanying intracranial dissection
- Local compression syndromes without ischemic events
- Concomitant diseases with increased bleeding risk

Adapted from Engelter ST, Brandt T, Debette S, et al. Antiplatelets versus anticoagulation in cervical artery dissection. Stroke 2007;38(9):2609.

the only prospective CAD series, in which none of 48 patients, followed for a mean of 7.8 years, had a recurrent dissection.[6]

Based on these observations—if anticoagulation is chosen as antithrombotic agent—it is mostly maintained for at least 3 to 6 months in a pragmatic approach. In the absence of ischemic events, (bleeding) complications, and major hemodynamic compromise at a 3-month or 6-month follow-up, aspirin may be used instead of anti-coagulants for another 6 to 9 months. Provided that (1) no first or recurrent ischemic event occurred under this regimen, (2) there is full restitution of the dissected artery on both MRI and neurosonography, and (3) there is no evidence of clinically silent ischemic lesions on MRI, stopping antithrombotic treatment may be considered. This decision should take into account the vascular risk profile, comorbidities, and patient perspective. The same criteria may be applied if antiplatelets rather than anti-coagulants were used as first antithrombotic treatment. In cases of development of an (asymptomatic) aneurysm at the site of the initially dissected artery (ie, a dissecting aneurysm), ongoing antiplatelet treatment is mostly preferred. This suggested approach is of unknown effectiveness (level U) and includes recommendations by other investigators[4,51,81,82] as well as from the authors' experiences.

ENDOVASCULAR TREATMENT

Although antithrombotic treatment has been sufficient in most patients, there are reports on endovascular treatment in CAD patients.[83–85] In most of the reported cases, endovascular treatment meant the use of angioplasty and stenting.[81,86,87] In their systematic review of endovascular stenting in extracranial CD and VAD, Pham and colleagues[86] identified 140 patients (153 arteries) with extracranial carotid dissection and 10 patients (12 arteries) with extracranial VAD. The technical success rate across all procedures was high (99% [ICAD] and 100% [extracranial VAD]). Periprocedural complications occurred in 1.3% (ICAD) and 0% (VAD), respectively. Carotid in-stent steno-occlusive complications were observed in 3 cases (3/150, 2%) and vertebral in-stent thrombosis was detected in 1 case (1/7, 14%). Within a mean follow-up period of 17.7 months (range 1–72 months), clinical complications occurred in 1.4% of all patients with carotid dissection. There were no clinical complications in the VAD group. In 70% of all reported cases, endovascular treatment was chosen because of the severity of the hemodynamic compromise with or without failure of the antithrombotic treatment or contraindications for the use of anticoagulants. Rupture of an extracranial dissecting aneurysm was another—however, rare—reported indication for stenting.[88] Thus, although endovascular treatment modalities seem relatively safe, it remains unclear if they are superior to antithrombotic treatment alone.

According to most investigators, endovascular treatment is usually reserved for CAD patients in whom antithrombotic therapy has failed, in particular in rapidly deteriorating patients or when hemodynamic infarction is impending, in ruptured dissecting aneurysm, or in iatrogenic CADs.[81,86–88]

SURGICAL TREATMENT

Current information on arterial surgery as treatment of CAD is scarce and most reports on surgery in CAD are older than 10 years. A systematic review across case series identified 135 ICAD patients who had arterial surgery. At the end of follow-up, 10 (7.4%) patients were reported dead and 7 (5.2%) "disabled." Furthermore, 7 ICAD patients (5.2%) suffered from stroke and 2 (1.5%) experienced ICH.[50] Thus, it seems that patients who had undergone surgery suffered from a higher rate of complications than those who received antithrombotic agents. This could be due to either treatment effects or to selection bias: patients who had surgery were initially more severely affected.[50] The latter is supported by the idea that surgery is typically reserved for complications, including severe, recurrently symptomatic stenosis or recurrent emboli.[89] Surgical treatment of CAD, however, carries risks of early occlusion, stroke, and cranial nerve injuries.[90] Hence, it has been suggested that surgery be limited to those cases of progression of symptoms in anatomically accessible lesions and patients for whom there are arguments against stenting.[89]

SUMMARY

CAD is a major cause of stroke in the young.[1] In most patients, CAD is confirmed by visualization of a mural hematoma. In this regard, MRI has a higher sensitivity than neurosonology but can be falsely negative in the very acute stage of CAD. The intramural blood accumulation should not be considered a reason to withhold IVT in patients with acute ischemic stroke associated with CAD. Acute endovascular treatment has been shown feasible. Current data do not provide any evidence that acute endovascular treatment is superior to IVT alone. Nevertheless, acute endovascular treatment is an alternative that is worthwhile studying further. Antiplatelets and anticoagulants are used to prevent stroke in CAD patients and there are arguments and counterarguments for either treatment strategy. The findings of 4 large meta-analyses across observational data do not suggest any superiority of either treatment approach. Three RCTs are under way and participation is encouraged to increase the level of evidence for the treatment of this important cause of stroke in the young. The available observational data suggest that in CAD patients angioplasty with stenting could be used in patients when antithrombotic therapy fails or hemodynamic infarction is impending. Surgery in such patients can be considered if there are arguments against angioplasty or stenting and the lesion is anatomically accessible.

REFERENCES

1. Yesilot Barlas N, Putaala J, Waje-Andreassen U, et al. Etiology of first-ever ischaemic stroke in European young adults: the 15 cities young stroke study. Eur J Neurol 2013;20(11):1431–9.
2. Leys DM, Stojkovic T, Begey S, et al. Follow-up of patients with history of cercial artery dissection. Cerebrovasc Dis 1995;5(1):7.
3. Leys D, Bandu L, Henon H, et al. Clinical outcome in 287 consecutive young adults (15 to 45 years) with ischemic stroke. Neurology 2002;59(1):26–33.
4. Debette S, Leys D. Cervical-artery dissections: predisposing factors, diagnosis, and outcome. Lancet Neurol 2009;8(7):668–78.
5. Nedeltchev K, der Maur TA, Georgiadis D, et al. Ischaemic stroke in young adults: predictors of outcome and recurrence. J Neurol Neurosurg Psychiatry 2005;76(2):191–5.
6. Lee VH, Brown RD Jr, Mandrekar JN, et al. Incidence and outcome of cervical artery dissection: a population-based study. Neurology 2006;67(10):1809–12.
7. Bejot Y, Daubail B, Debette S, et al. Incidence and outcome of cerebrovascular events related to cervical artery dissection: the Dijon Stroke Registry. Int J Stroke 2014;9(7):879–82.
8. Schievink WI, Mokri B, Whisnant JP. Internal carotid artery dissection in a community. Rochester, Minnesota, 1987–1992. Stroke 1993;24(11):1678–80.
9. Giroud M, Fayolle H, Andre N, et al. Incidence of internal carotid artery dissection in the community of Dijon. J Neurol Neurosurg Psychiatry 1994;57(11):1443.

10. Debette S, Metso TM, Pezzini A, et al. CADISP-genetics: an International project searching for genetic risk factors of cervical artery dissections. Int J Stroke 2009; 4(3):224–30.
11. Debette S, Grond-Ginsbach C, Bodenant M, et al. Differential features of carotid and vertebral artery dissections: the CADISP study. Neurology 2011;77(12): 1174–81.
12. Beletsky V, Nadareishvili Z, Lynch J, et al. Cervical arterial dissection: time for a therapeutic trial? Stroke 2003;34(12):2856–60.
13. Engelter ST, Lyrer PA, Kirsch EC, et al. Long-term follow-up after extracranial internal carotid artery dissection. Eur Neurol 2000;44(4):199–204.
14. Arnold M, Kappeler L, Georgiadis D, et al. Gender differences in spontaneous cervical artery dissection. Neurology 2006;67(6):1050–2.
15. Georgiadis D, Arnold M, von Buedingen HC, et al. Aspirin vs anticoagulation in carotid artery dissection: a study of 298 patients. Neurology 2009;72(21):1810–5.
16. Metso TM, Debette S, Grond-Ginsbach C, et al. Age-dependent differences in cervical artery dissection. J Neurol 2012;259(10):2202–10.
17. Brandt T, Caplan L. Spontaneous arterial dissection. Curr Treat Options Neurol 2001;3(5):463–9.
18. Touze E, Gauvrit JY, Moulin T, et al. Risk of stroke and recurrent dissection after a cervical artery dissection: a multicenter study. Neurology 2003;61(10):1347–51.
19. Metso AJ, Metso TM, Debette S, et al. Gender and cervical artery dissection. Eur J Neurol 2012;19(4):594–602.
20. Engelter ST, Brandt T, Debette S, et al. Antiplatelets versus anticoagulation in cervical artery dissection. Stroke 2007;38(9):2605–11.
21. Engelter ST, Grond-Ginsbach C, Metso TM, et al. Cervical artery dissection: trauma and other potential mechanical trigger events. Neurology 2013;80(21): 1950–7.
22. Schievink WI. Spontaneous dissection of the carotid and vertebral arteries. N Engl J Med 2001;344(12):898–906.
23. Arnold M, Nedeltchev K, Sturzenegger M, et al. Thrombolysis in patients with acute stroke caused by cervical artery dissection: analysis of 9 patients and review of the literature. Arch Neurol 2002;59(4):549–53.
24. Engelter ST, Rutgers MP, Hatz F, et al. Intravenous thrombolysis in stroke attributable to cervical artery dissection. Stroke 2009;40(12):3772–6.
25. Fluri F, Lyrer PA, Steck AJ, et al. Internal carotid artery dissection with occlusion during heparing therapy. Schweiz Arch Neurol Psychiatr 2007;158(7):3.
26. Nebelsieck J, Sengelhoff C, Nassenstein I, et al. Sensitivity of neurovascular ultrasound for the detection of spontaneous cervical artery dissection. J Clin Neurosci 2009;16(1):79–82.
27. Engelter ST, Dallongeville J, Kloss M, et al. Thrombolysis in cervical artery dissection–data from the Cervical Artery Dissection and Ischaemic Stroke Patients (CADISP) database. Eur J Neurol 2012;19(9):1199–206.
28. Kamp TJ, Goldschmidt-Clermont PJ, Brinker JA, et al. Myocardial infarction, aortic dissection, and thrombolytic therapy. Am Heart J 1994;128(6 Pt 1):1234–7.
29. Lee CH, Lim J. Type A aortic dissection: a hidden and lethal cause for failed thrombolytic treatment in acute myocardial infarction. Heart 2007;93(7):825.
30. Delgado MG, Garcia R, Murias E. Is intravenous thrombolysis useful in carotid artery dissection with tandem occlusion? J Stroke Cerebrovasc Dis 2012;21(1):87–8.
31. Linfante I, Llinas RH, Selim M, et al. Clinical and vascular outcome in internal carotid artery versus middle cerebral artery occlusions after intravenous tissue plasminogen activator. Stroke 2002;33(8):2066–71.

32. Ahmed N, Wahlgren N, Grond M, et al. Implementation and outcome of thrombolysis with alteplase 3-4.5 h after an acute stroke: an updated analysis from SITS-ISTR. Lancet Neurol 2010;9(9):866–74.
33. Zinkstok SM, Vergouwen MD, Engelter ST, et al. Safety and functional outcome of thrombolysis in dissection-related ischemic stroke: a meta-analysis of individual patient data. Stroke 2011;42(9):2515–20.
34. Fuentes B, Masjuán J, Egido J, et al. Is intravenous TPA treatment beneficial in acute ischemic stroke related to internal carotid dissection. Cerebrovasc Dis 2007;(Suppl 2) [abstract: 23]:108.
35. Rudolf J, Neveling M, Grond M, et al. Stroke following internal carotid artery occlusion - a contra-indication for intravenous thrombolysis? Eur J Neurol 1999; 6(1):51–5.
36. Derex L, Nighoghossian N, Turjman F, et al. Intravenous tPA in acute ischemic stroke related to internal carotid artery dissection. Neurology 2000;54(11): 2159–61.
37. Georgiadis D, Lanczik O, Schwab S, et al. IV thrombolysis in patients with acute stroke due to spontaneous carotid dissection. Neurology 2005;64(9): 1612–4.
38. Tissue plasminogen activator for acute ischemic stroke. The National Institute of Neurological Disorders and Stroke rt-PA Stroke Study Group. N Engl J Med 1995; 333(24):1581–7.
39. Hacke W, Kaste M, Bluhmki E, et al. Thrombolysis with alteplase 3 to 4.5 hours after acute ischemic stroke. N Engl J Med 2008;359(13):1317–29.
40. Lavallee PC, Mazighi M, Saint-Maurice JP, et al. Stent-assisted endovascular thrombolysis versus intravenous thrombolysis in internal carotid artery dissection with tandem internal carotid and middle cerebral artery occlusion. Stroke 2007; 38(8):2270–4.
41. Lekoubou A, Cho TH, Nighoghossian N, et al. Combined intravenous recombinant-tissular plasminogen activator and endovascular treatment of spontaneous occlusive internal carotid dissection with tandem intracranial artery occlusion. Eur Neurol 2010;63(4):211–4.
42. Baumgartner RW, Georgiadis D, Nedeltchev K, et al. Stent-assisted endovascular thrombolysis versus intravenous thrombolysis in internal carotid artery dissection with tandem internal carotid and middle cerebral artery occlusion. Stroke 2008;39(2):e27–8.
43. Vergouwen MD, Beentjes PA, Nederkoorn PJ. Thrombolysis in patients with acute ischemic stroke due to arterial extracranial dissection. Eur J Neurol 2009;16(5): 646–9.
44. Mourand I, Brunel H, Vendrell JF, et al. Endovascular stent-assisted thrombolysis in acute occlusive carotid artery dissection. Neuroradiology 2010;52(2): 135–40.
45. Broderick JP, Palesch YY, Demchuk AM, et al. Endovascular therapy after intravenous t-PA versus t-PA alone for stroke. N Engl J Med 2013;368(10): 893–903.
46. Weimar C, Kraywinkel K, Hagemeister C, et al. Recurrent stroke after cervical artery dissection. J Neurol Neurosurg Psychiatry 2010;81(8):869–73.
47. Kennedy F, Lanfranconi S, Hicks C, et al. Antiplatelets vs anticoagulation for dissection: CADISS nonrandomized arm and meta-analysis. Neurology 2012; 79(7):686–9.
48. Lyrer P, Engelter S. Antithrombotic drugs for carotid artery dissection. Cochrane Database Syst Rev 2010;(10):CD000255.

49. Gensicke H, Ahlhelm F, Jung S, et al. New ischemic brain lesions in cervical artery dissection stratified to antiplatelets or anticoagulants. Eur J Neurol 2015. (in press).
50. Lyrer P, Engelter S. Antithrombotic drugs for carotid artery dissection. Cochrane Database Syst Rev 2003;(3):CD000255.
51. Arnold M, Fischer U, Bousser MG. Treatment issues in spontaneous cervicocephalic artery dissections. Int J Stroke 2011;6(3):213–8.
52. Menon RK, Markus HS, Norris JW. Results of a UK questionnaire of diagnosis and treatment in cervical artery dissection. J Neurol Neurosurg Psychiatry 2008;79(5):612.
53. Donnan GA, Davis SM. Extracranial arterial dissection: anticoagulation is the treatment of choice. Stroke 2005;36(9):2043–4.
54. Lyrer PA. Extracranial arterial dissection: anticoagulation is the treatment of choice: against. Stroke 2005;36(9):2042–3.
55. Norris JW. Extracranial arterial dissection: anticoagulation is the treatment of choice: for. Stroke 2005;36(9):2041–2.
56. Menon R, Kerry S, Norris JW, et al. Treatment of cervical artery dissection: a systematic review and meta-analysis. J Neurol Neurosurg Psychiatry 2008;79(10): 1122–7.
57. Sarikaya H, da Costa BR, Baumgartner RW, et al. Antiplatelets versus anticoagulants for the treatment of cervical artery dissection: Bayesian meta-analysis. PLoS One 2013;8(9):e72697.
58. Bonati LH, Jongen LM, Haller S, et al. New ischaemic brain lesions on MRI after stenting or endarterectomy for symptomatic carotid stenosis: a substudy of the International Carotid Stenting Study (ICSS). Lancet Neurol 2010;9(4):353–62.
59. Bonati LH, Lyrer PA, Fluri F. Cerebral microbleeds after carotid revascularization - a prospective MRI study. Cerebrovasc Dis 2008;(Supply 2) [abstract]:55.
60. Droste DW, Junker K, Stogbauer F, et al. Clinically silent circulating microemboli in 20 patients with carotid or vertebral artery dissection. Cerebrovasc Dis 2001; 12(3):181–5.
61. Srinivasan J, Newell DW, Sturzenegger M, et al. Transcranial Doppler in the evaluation of internal carotid artery dissection. Stroke 1996;27(7):1226–30.
62. Koennecke HC, Trocio SH Jr, Mast H, et al. Microemboli on transcranial Doppler in patients with spontaneous carotid artery dissection. J Neuroimaging 1997;7(4):217–20.
63. Molina CA, Alvarez-Sabin J, Schonewille W, et al. Cerebral microembolism in acute spontaneous internal carotid artery dissection. Neurology 2000;55(11):1738–40.
64. Oliveira V, Batista P, Soares F, et al. HITS in internal carotid dissections. Cerebrovasc Dis 2001;11(4):330–4.
65. Goertler M, Blaser T, Krueger S, et al. Cessation of embolic signals after antithrombotic prevention is related to reduced risk of recurrent arterioembolic transient ischaemic attack and stroke. J Neurol Neurosurg Psychiatry 2002;72(3): 338–42.
66. Markus HS, Droste DW, Kaps M, et al. Dual antiplatelet therapy with clopidogrel and aspirin in symptomatic carotid stenosis evaluated using doppler embolic signal detection: the Clopidogrel and Aspirin for Reduction of Emboli in Symptomatic Carotid Stenosis (CARESS) trial. Circulation 2005;111(17):2233–40.
67. Perren F, Bocquet L, Saulnier F, et al. Does anticoagulation harm in acute cervical artery dissection? Cerebrovasc Dis 2006;21(Suppl 4) [abstract]:146.
68. Machet A, Fonseca AC, Oppenheim C, et al. Does anticoagulation promote mural hematoma growth or delayed occlusion in spontaneous cervical artery dissections? Cerebrovasc Dis 2013;35(2):175–81.

69. Dreier JP, Lurtzing F, Kappmeier M, et al. Delayed occlusion after internal carotid artery dissection under heparin. Cerebrovasc Dis 2004;18(4):296–303.

70. Bachmann R, Nassenstein I, Kooijman H, et al. High-resolution magnetic resonance imaging (MRI) at 3.0 Tesla in the short-term follow-up of patients with proven cervical artery dissection. Invest Radiol 2007;42(6):460–6.

71. Combe J, Poinsard P, Besancenot J, et al. Free-floating thrombus of the extracranial internal carotid artery. Ann Vasc Surg 1990;4(6):558–62.

72. Ast G, Woimant F, Georges B, et al. Spontaneous dissection of the internal carotid artery in 68 patients. Eur J Med 1993;2(8):466–72.

73. Steinke W, Rautenberg W, Schwartz A, et al. Noninvasive monitoring of internal carotid artery dissection. Stroke 1994;25(5):998–1005.

74. Brandt T, Stoegbauer F, Ringelstein EB, et al. Dissektion hirnversorgender Arterien. In: Diener HC, Hacke W, Forsting M, editors. Schlaganfall: Referenzreihe Neurologie-Klinische Neurologie. 1st edition. NewYork: Thieme; 2004. p. 176–81.

75. Investigators TOAST-Study. Low molecular weight heparinoid, ORG 10172 (danaparoid), and outcome after acute ischemic stroke: a randomized controlled trial. The Publications Committee for the Trial of ORG 10172 in Acute Stroke Treatment (TOAST) Investigators. JAMA 1998;279(16):1265–72.

76. Adams HP Jr, Adams RJ, Brott T, et al. Guidelines for the early management of patients with ischemic stroke: a scientific statement from the Stroke Council of the American Stroke Association. Stroke 2003;34(4):1056–83.

77. Nedeltchev K, Bickel S, Arnold M, et al. R2-recanalization of spontaneous carotid artery dissection. Stroke 2009;40(2):499–504.

78. Baracchini C, Tonello S, Meneghetti G, et al. Neurosonographic monitoring of 105 spontaneous cervical artery dissections: a prospective study. Neurology 2010; 75(21):1864–70.

79. Kremer C, Mosso M, Georgiadis D, et al. Carotid dissection with permanent and transient occlusion or severe stenosis: long-term outcome. Neurology 2003; 60(2):271–5.

80. Dittrich R, Nassenstein I, Bachmann R, et al. Polyarterial clustered recurrence of cervical artery dissection seems to be the rule. Neurology 2007;69(2):180–6.

81. Rahme RJ, Aoun SG, McClendon J Jr, et al. Spontaneous cervical and cerebral arterial dissections: diagnosis and management. Neuroimaging Clin N Am 2013; 23(4):661–71.

82. German Society of Neurology [Deutsche Gesellschaft für Neurologie]. Spontane Dissektionen der extrakraniellen und intrakraniellen hirnversorgenden Arterien. Leitlinien für Diagnostik und Therapie in der Neurologie. 2012 2012;IL_24_2012(AWMF-Registernummer: 030/005):9. Available at: http://www.dgn.org/leitlinien-online-2012/inhalte-nach-kapitel/2313-ll-24-2012-spontane-dissektionen-der-extrakraniellen-und-intrakraniellen-hirnversorgenden-arterien.html. Accessed September 29, 2014.

83. Edgell RC, Abou-Chebl A, Yadav JS. Endovascular management of spontaneous carotid artery dissection. J Vasc Surg 2005;42(5):854–60 [discussion: 860].

84. Fava M, Meneses L, Loyola S, et al. Carotid artery dissection: endovascular treatment. Report of 12 patients. Catheter Cardiovasc Interv 2008;71(5):694–700.

85. Assadian A, Senekowitsch C, Rotter R, et al. Long-term results of covered stent repair of internal carotid artery dissections. J Vasc Surg 2004;40(3):484–7.

86. Pham MH, Rahme RJ, Arnaout O, et al. Endovascular stenting of extracranial carotid and vertebral artery dissections: a systematic review of the literature. Neurosurgery 2011;68(4):856–66 [discussion: 866].

87. Ahlhelm F, Benz RM, Ulmer S, et al. Endovascular treatment of cervical artery dissection: ten case reports and review of the literature. Interv Neurol 2013; 1(3–4):143–50.
88. Goyal MS, Derdeyn CP. The diagnosis and management of supraaortic arterial dissections. Curr Opin Neurol 2009;22(1):80–9.
89. Rao AS, Makaroun MS, Marone LK, et al. Long-term outcomes of internal carotid artery dissection. J Vasc Surg 2011;54(2):370–4 [discussion: 375].
90. Muller BT, Luther B, Hort W, et al. Surgical treatment of 50 carotid dissections: indications and results. J Vasc Surg 2000;31(5):980–8.